PaleoJay's Smoothie Cafe

by Jay P. Bowers

PaleoJay's Smoothie Cafe!

CONTENTS

DEDICATION

To Abram Gustafson

Grandson, and hope for the future

FOREWORD

Perhaps you wonder- why another book about the Paleo diet? Haven't there been many books released, especially in the past couple of years that are supposedly the same thing, albeit maybe a little "different color" in a few aspects?

Yes, and yes.

The difference between those and what you now hold in our hands is that this is a guide that brings it all together, with diet, lifestyle, and exercise- and all in a very accessible and useable manner!

The green smoothie as a foundational aspect of the Paleo diet has not been a popular idea within the movement, until very recently. It is KEY to achieving the maximum results in nutrition, especially in this modern age of nutrient depleted soils, and incredibly busy lives with less free time than ever.

This is why I call it a Paleo Green Smoothie- since over time I have researched and tried this and added that, until I have come up with a pretty much perfect nutritional powerhouse.

PaleoJay's Smoothie Cafe!

***

Add it to your regimen, along with all else that I recommend here at PaleoJay's Smoothie Cafe, and I predict a very healthy, slim and defined, strong and vital YOU!

Welcome to the Cafe!

PaleoJay

Why Paleo?

WHY PALEO DIET?

Why should you adopt the Paleo Diet? Well, let's say this is your goal: To get healthy, lean and very fit. To be completely disease and symptom free for your entire life without gradual deterioration, and stay happy and productive!

I'm sure anyone would agree that such an outcome would be wonderful! Perhaps you hardly know where to start though...

I can absolutely guarantee that if you will change the way you eat to be more in accordance with our evolutionary heritage, or the way we have adapted to the natural world, you will be MUCH healthier, MUCH leaner, and much HAPPIER than you are right now! And I maintain that you can make these changes, and reap these fantastic results no matter how old or young you are, no matter what shape you are in now, and that these changes will happen quite rapidly as well!

Ready to get started?

You just have to need to want to make these changes! Certain bad foods will need to be eliminated from your diet, and hopefully also the diets of your family members as well. Wouldn't it be great if not only YOU were healthy and happy for your lifetime, but if your spouse and children were as well??

It can happen, and again, it can happen relatively quickly too.
Most people object to doing new things because of a perception that it will "cost too much" or that it will "take too much time". Your new paleo lifestyle will do neither of those things, but will instead save you money by

#

PALEO DIET TO LOSE FAT

The Paleo Diet has shown remarkable success in helping people to lose fat/weight, and achieve a much better "body composition". The amazing thing is that it can bring these changes about without:

1. Hunger
2. Long sessions of exercise
3. Injury from those long, boring exercise sessions you thought were necessary

Really! But how can this be?

It's really just simple, proven science!
aAmerica. Wheat is now completely genetically modified to the point where it has no similarity to the ancient wheat of the Bible, or even to the wheat from the 1960's!!
This is a huge point: if you wish to research the topic in depth, I refer you to the book Wheat Belly by William Davis.

But, since all carbohydrates, like wheat, corn, white potatoes, etc. turns to sugar in the body, that is more than enough reason alone to severely limit them in the diet.

The other thing to limit greatly in your diet is SUGAR.

When you eat sugar, or its twin- carbohydrates- your body responds to the rise in blood sugar, (which is actually an emergency situation for your body!), by producing massive quantities of insulin. Insulin, which as we know is what Type 2 (self-induced) Diabetics lose the ability to produce, after many years of ingesting so much sugar/carbohydrates that their body has become overwhelmed by the bodily insult! Don't let this happen to you- it is becoming

#

IF YOU DON'T EAT PALEO YOU ARE PROBABLY NUTRIENT DEFICIENT!

I hope that title got your attention, because it's true- if you eat any sort of S.A.D. standard American diet, or even any type of vegan, vegetarian, or even the so-called Mediterranean diet- you are deficient in vital nutrients!

You probably get too many calories, but very little in the way of actual, health sustaining and health building nutrients- the result is inevitably going to be

Constant hunger
Blood sugar spikes and dips
Feelings of brain fog, depression, and anxiety
Progressive extreme weakness as you age, inability to sleep
Obesity and skin problems
Eventual crippling disease

I really don't mean to scare you, but if I do a little, that can only help to scare you into changing your diet and lifestyle! It really isn't that hard, especially for all of the rewards your health will enjoy, but there are are few things that are almost universal for modern Americans:

Leaky gut- this is the big one, and the hardest one. You really must get away from grains, primarily wheat and its built in poison gluten. This one thing, wheat, which is the most consumed food in the modern day, has been bred into a Frankenstein monster, and is by itself setting us up for all sorts of autoimmune diseases. Get rid of wheat, and you are really more than half way there! (Incidentally, this is the only real difference between the highly thought of Mediterranean diet and the paleo diet, since both modes of eating encourage real foods like butter and oils, lots of green plant foods, and lots of herbs and spices). But, this is a really crucial difference!

Get some magnesium into your diet- magnesium deficiency is pandemic in these modern times. The very best way is to start including green leafy vegetables into your diet in a big way! The very best and most effective way to accomplish that is by buying a Vitamix blender, and making a green Paleo smoothie to drink daily- it doesn't have to be big- I fill Ball 16 oz. canning jars, and fill about 5 from each smoothie blending canister! Then, I just take out one each day, and enjoy it for breakfast, along with my eggs and bacon and coffee mixed with a little coconut oil and cream. That one action will yield the most bang for the buck- go to www.paleojay.com and click on the Vitamix link, and you can order one direct from Vitamix. Get that magnesium back into your cells; here's the negative reasons why s deficiency matters:

Neurological:

Behavioral disturbances
Irritability and anxiety
Lethargy
Impaired memory and cognitive function
Anorexia or loss of appetite
Nausea and vomiting
Seizures
Muscular:
Weakness
Muscle spasms (tetany)
Tics

Muscle cramps
Hyperactive reflexes
Impaired muscle coordination (ataxia)
Tremors
Involuntary eye movements and vertigo
Difficulty swallowing

Metabolic:

Increased intracellular calcium
Hyperglycemia
Calcium deficiency
Potassium deficiency
Cardiovascular:
Irregular or rapid heartbeat
Coronary spasms
Among children:
Growth retardation or "failure to thrive"

CONDITIONS RELATED TO PROBLEMS OF MAGNESIUM

In addition to symptoms of overt hypomagnesemia
(clinically low serum magnesium), the following conditions
represent possible indicators of chronic latent magnesium
deficiency

Depression
Chronic fatigue syndrome
ADHD
Epilepsy
Parkinson's disease
Sleep problems
Migraine
Cluster headaches
Osteoporosis
Premenstrual syndrome

Chest pain (angina)
Cardiac arrhythmias
Coronary artery disease and atherosclerosis
Hypertension
Type II diabetes
Asthma

And clean up the rest of your diet- cut the sugar way, way back! A few empty carbs are OK from time to time, like gluten free baked goods and gluten free pizza crust, but make it rare- they just turn to sugar with no nutrients attached! Try to eat nutrient dense foods- grass fed meats, wild caught seafoods, sweet potatoes and white potatoes (don't eat the skin! loaded with anti-nutrients!), and white rice in moderation. Occasional corn chips appear to be fine for most active people, as does occasional popcorn topped with real pastured butter and sea salt! But keep the carbs down; Americans have come to be carboholics, hence their incredible increase in girth and disease over the past 50 years or so.

One more option you may want to consider for magnesium (it is that important I keep coming back to it!) is ancient minerals.

This is a concentrated form of magnesium, completely uncontaminated since it is drawn from dead sea sources well below the surface of the earth! You can either rub it on your skin as a lotion or spray it on your skin, and it is absorbed into the body without having to pass through the digestive system- I have used it on people with all sorts of cramps and restless leg syndromes and it works like a charm! A good way to "kick start" your magnesium up to normal levels while you change your diet to keep them up from day to day.

What else? Glad you asked, grasshopper!

*＊＊

Get some exercise- park far away, and walk where you are going. Stretch each morning, and do some Perfectly Paleo Exercise each day to get started! Walk barefoot on the earth, get out into the sun, and rejuvenate yourself in nature as often as you can. Your Vitamin D levels are the next most important thing to take care of! So get out into the sunshine for at least 15 minutes each day, and a good supplement can help there as well. Get a liquid vitamin D is the most efficient; just add a few drops to your green paleo smoothie!

So there it is- a simple recipe for total health and wellness! It's not that hard, it's not complicated, and it is very, very effective!

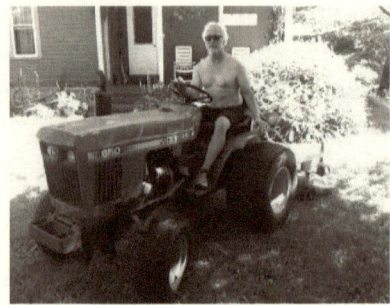

#

Go Paleo Now- Before you are SICK!

I really hope you listen to me on this! Well, actually, I always hope you'll listen to me, but this is rather crucial.
It is an all-too-common scenario:

Someone gets sick! I mean really, auto-immune disease, cancer or heart disease, diabetes or another Paleo diet preventable disease sick...

＊＊＊

THEN they come around, in desperation, eventually and after lots of searching and research and usually after trying out the drugs and surgeries that conventional medicine offers for their disease (or diseases).

While late is better than never to discover the paleo type of ancestral diet and all the health benefits and just better way of life that it offers; well, once you already are sick, it might not be enough!

Let me put it this way- once you have put in decade upon decade of bad eating and living habits, like not getting enough sleep, being overstressed on a regular basis, not maintaining your "tribe" of good friends and family, church fellow members, and others you are "connected" with, and neglecting to exercise naturally and getting out into nature and the sunshine....

That is one deep hole to dig out of! Your body will undoubtedly be wracked with inflammation, have a really poor gut microbe set, and will in many ways be the equivalent of a car that has been run at high speeds, with low, dirty oil, and without proper maintenance. It is prone to one or more serious, life-altering diseases to emerge at any time!

Let me offer a solution! Start following the Paleo Prescription as soon as possible! The earlier you adopt it, the less damage you will do to your precious body (and mind!). That's another thing: the mind is every bit as susceptible to a bad SAD Standard American Diet of processed crap foods as the body. Can you say Alzheimer's?

Look up the particulars of the Paleo Diet! The internet is good www.paleojay.com has lots of information, but so does www.RobbWolfe.com, www.ChrisKresser.com, and Loren

Cordain on
thepaleodiet.com.

There are also great books on the subject: The Paleo Solution by Robb Wolf is great, and my own Perfectly Paleo Exercise ebook is very accessible- there are others. Oh yes, Neanderthin by Ray Audette was published in 1999, making it ancient by Paleo standards, but it is spot on still! And for the grand daddy of them all, there is always Weston A. Price's 1939 book Nutrition and Physical Degeneration, which is pretty much pure genius- there is still a widely active Weston A Price foundation throughout the world, celebrating what he discovered way back then!

So, there is no dearth of information, far from it. Just get started on the basics, which pretty much all practitioners agree on:

Eliminate processed foods- fast foods, fake foods like vegetable oils and margarine, modern grains like wheat, baked goods and cereals, and most sugar.

Eat LOTS of green veggies, cruciferous veggies, some berries, spices, fermented foods- in other words, just eat real foods!

Start to lead the healthiest, most satisfying life there is; the life God and nature intended for us, the one we evolved to thrive in-

The Ancestral, Paleo type of diet, exercise, tribal connection, and living as naturally in the world as we possibly can in this modern age.

Anything else is not just an invitation to disease and "physical degeneration" as Weston A. Price discovered...it is really a recipe for a sad life in general!

#

OUR CHILDREN ARE THE CANARIES IN THE COAL MINE

I'm afraid that this sad fact is the truth- our children in America, and increasingly world wide, are suffering at ever earlier ages under the scourge of

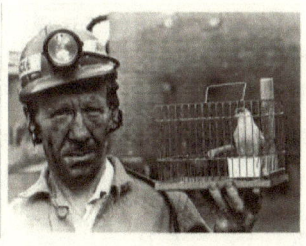

autoimmune conditions.

I have been witnessing this process for years now; I have been paleo for about 10 years or so now. I have evolved, and slowly added in more good things (like better exercise, higher quality food, better sleep and meditation), and benefited greatly! I am now 63 years of age, and in far better shape than I was at 50: no more painful joints, knee or shoulder pain (from weight lifting, running, and an inflammatory diet). No more migraine headaches (primarily, I found out, from gluten- when I eliminated gluten and in fact most grains altogether, I never got another headache again. I threw away my pharmaceutical medicine...

* * *

On the other hand, most of my friends and peers, who are mostly in the 40 - 60 year age bracket, have picked up numerous diseases and conditions. Diabetes and "diabesity", of which the second predicts the former have happened to many, along with heart disease, gerd, acid reflux, sleep apnea and snoring, and even some cancer. And the list goes on...

These are the ones who do not listen to my advice. They eat the standard American diet of pizza, fast foods, processed crap, bread and pasta. Most try to "cut their fat intake" by switching exclusively away from butter and full fat dairy, and try to "cut calories" by drinking skim milk, and cereal for breakfast, along with "healthy whole grain toast" with margarine on top.

Almost all of them are on statins, against my arguments about it's uselessness and extreme danger. Many dose themselves almost daily with high doses of aspirin, tylenol and ibuprofen to deal with their many aches and pains. Exercise? They walk at the mall...

Those that have followed my lead are about as healthy as I am! Many have reversed conditions like diabetes (type 2), skin conditions like eczema and psoriasis, and all sorts of digestive ailments. Most don't exercise nearly as much, but they have had wonderful results, healthwise, regardless!

But they are the older generation, on their way out. What is troubling me now, is that all of the diseases that my middle-aged friends have are now turning up in children I have known since birth!

Type one diabetes in 13 year olds to 30 year olds. Diverticulitis, Arthritis, hasimotos, and infertility, Hashimoto thyroiditis, type I diabetes, lupus, and vasculitis. It is starting to run rampant among young people, this taking them down by having their own immune system attacking their very own body! Why? And why is this new? This stuff didn't happen, or very, very rarely in my generation when we were young. Now it hits younger and younger people, in more and more numbers! When I was young, in the 1950's, it really was like the movie Back to the Future. Families ate at home, things like pot roast and vegetables, everyone got plenty of sleep before school, high fructose corn syrup had not been invented yet, and pesticides and herbicide use was very little. Most meat was raised on small farms, and was pastured on grass, not corn. There was the local "malt shop", but this was just for high school socializing and things like sodas and milkshakes, real ones, which are a far cry from the chemical laden, crap-meat fast food in most fast food joints today!

Fast forward to today, or even to 30 years ago: increasingly BOTH parents have to work, primarily to pay the TAXES that have escalated in this country. Now, there is no "home maker" to make the nutritious, healthy, home cooked quality meals anymore. The parents just rush the kids to a fast food joint, and buy them corn syrup or (worse) artificially sweetened soft drinks, fries cooked in vegetable oil, and gluten covered crap grain fed meat covered in sugar (ketchup) and mayo (vegetable crap oil)... day after day after day after day...
Then, when the mom does actually have time to cook, like on weekends, she buys those biscuits in tubes, and canned cheap soups, and other processed foods, throwing them together in quick recipes that make a gluten sugar bomb of a meal... over and over and over again! And then, for a change, they order pizza!

10 to 20 years of this, and your gut lining is leaky and destroyed. Toxins from this bad food, and actually from

21

anywhere that get into your digestive system and have nothing to stop them- they go right into your bloodstream!

At this point, your immune system can hardly tell the difference between your own bodily cells, and all of these invaders- it goes into maximum fight response! And it winds up attacking your own bodily parts- your digestive system is often the first to be attacked, since it is right there. (Diverticulitis, Crohn's disease)

But, it can go anywhere- attacking your joints (arthritis), your pancreas (Type 1 diabetes), your skin (eczema or psoriasis), or your thyroid. (Hashimoto's disease) It can even result in your own immune system attacking your brain. This, I believe, could be one reason for the huge increase in autism, severe mood disorders like depression, and many other behavior problems in children today!

And so, where does that leave us?
The state of nutrition and lifestyle in America today has reached a low ebb. From the very hard, physical, yet nutrient richness of our great grandfathers and grandmothers we have come to this- the world of Wall.E.

If you have never seen this Disney movie from 2008, I recommend you do. It pretty much depicts where we are headed: Wall-E shows a future human race that is so lazy and decrepit that everyone just rides around all day in little electric carts, and drinking soft drinks from giant cups as they go all day. Robots do everything for them, and all they do is to...barely exist! Seemed so far-fetched just 7 years ago, and now- it seems like we are half way there!

Remember my analogy in the title of this podcast?

Our children are our canaries in the coal mine!

* * *

If you are not aware, many years ago, coal miners would let down a basket of canaries into a coal mine shaft to determine if it was safe to breathe the air down there. If they pulled up the basket by the rope, and the canaries were dead, or really sick, they knew they could not yet send humans down.

Our children are sick. They are OUR CANARIES!

#

BEGINNING PALEO DIET!

Maybe you've just been hearing about this "paleo diet" thing, or maybe you have a friend or know someone who has had amazing results from eating and living according to this template...

Perhaps you have tried to ignore the whole thing, not wanting to change your life and mindset around after all these years of being brainwashed into the low fat high carb Standard American Diet LIE...

But, since the ancestral diet and it's benefits are very real, and the path we are on in the Western world is leading us into slow suicide by eating ourselves into diabesity, accompanied by prescriptions of pharmaceutical drugs that compromise our health even more with all of the inevitable side effects, resulting in early disability and death- well, "going Paleo" starts to not sound that hard after all!

So, how do you finally get off the sidelines and start making meaningful, healing change??

Clean out your cupboards! Ditch the grains- bread, pancake mixes, brownie mixes, cereals, vegetable and soy oils, Crisco, anything you have that is not real food. If it's not in your

23

house, you won't eat it.

Try a Paleo smoothie! This is a pet project of mine- I have developed my smoothie into a drink that is continually evolving, since I want to maximize my nutrition optimally, but starting out, keep it simple:

Just get out your standard, $20 blender, and make a simple Paleo Smoothie:

1 can of coconut milk

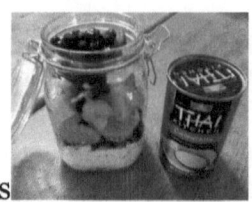

handful of fresh strawberries

a big leaf of fresh kale
a banana
sprinkle of cinnamon

Blend it all together for about a minute or so- you're done!

Easy, right? It's so easy, you will start to think as I did- "Hey, what if I add this ingredient, and that other super healthy food, and then that..."

You are on the slippery slope to health my friend, and trust me, that's where you want to be! You'll start adding raw eggs, and then you'll want the convenience of using frozen vegetables, and the ability to mix just about anything, smoothly and easily into your smoothies- at that point you'll want to get a Vitamix blender, since it it the best tool for engineering the most amazingly healthy and filling and appetizing Paleo smoothies on the planet!

PaleoJay's Smoothie Cafe!

Interestingly, I just read a news story in Barron's, the business newspaper, detailing how the Starbucks chain has bought a smoothie making chain of restaurants, and plans to expand dramatically, doing for smoothies what they have already done for coffee! While I'm sure it's better than the unhealthy coffee drink market they've been profiting from at the expense of the American people's health, I would suggest strongly that you make your own! I guarantee that anything made by a corporate giant will be vastly inferior, since the bottom line for such a company is to cut costs wherever possible, to maximize profits. This means low quality ingredients, cheaper, faster, worser! (There, I invented a word!)

So, Go Paleo Young Man! (Or woman)!

At first, I would just make a smoothie each morning, and eat eggs and meat, salads, seafood, veggies and nuts with a little fruit sometimes. For me, cheese and whole cream are fine-try them out, if you feel worse, maybe they aren't for you!
 Some folks can handle dairy, some can't... raw dairy is vastly preferable, if available.

Believe it or not, at first I do not recommend any exercise!
 Especially, if your are a "cardio-holic", used to doing lots of running, bicycling, aerobics, etc. just stop for awhile!
 Getting your diet in order is far more important than exercise, and along with adequate sleep each night of 8 hours or better, will get you 90% where you want to go. Just concentrate on those things for a month- learn to eat, and sleep like a paleolithic hunter-gatherer.   Next month we'll add in exercise- hey, I even have an eBook specifically about it...

A good idea, especially if you currently have health problems, would be to have a blood work up just before starting this at

25

the Doctor's office. Then, a month later, have it done again. I guarantee the results will startle both you and your Doctor- and then, he'll probably try to talk you out of doing something so "crazy"...

The thing to remember is this- even if all you had read about nutrition was this one blog, you would already know more about nutrition than your Doctor learned in all of medical school. So, take his or her opinions with more than a grain of good sea salt...

After your initial month, take a good look at how you look, how clearly you can think,and how you feel. Perhaps you already have had some drastic changes; many people do. And after actually sticking to the diet for one month, almost no one goes back to their standard diet! The benefits are that compelling- you may even become like me, shouting the news from the rooftops, because you almost can't believe the benefits of eating real food like a real person!

There is more to learn, in fact you never learn it all- but just do this for a month first- no need to rush things!

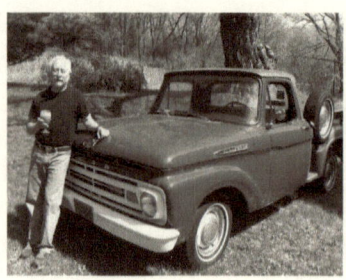

\#

BE A NEW PALEO YOU- GO BACK TO THE FUTURE!

* * *

Yes, you really can become the New Paleo You! It won't happen overnight, but considering that you've been sliding into the Old Neolithic you for decades, at least, you will be very pleased to hear that your new self, no matter how much you've been damaged metabolically from bad nutrition and exercise advice, is only months away in most cases.

Let's take a bad case as an example- let's say you are a life-long exerciser, mainly running and other forms of "cardio" or "aerobics" like spinning classes, dance classes, jazzercise, whatever kind of exercise that only is supposed to burn calories and help endurance... this kind of exercise is really bad! just so you know, it is counterproductive, and will only teach your body to hold onto fat, raise your cortisol or stress hormones, lower your immunity to colds and flu, and wear out your joints.

And let's say you have been a "yo-yo" dieter for years- reducing calories to 1500 per day or less, losing weight (not only fat, but mostly muscle first, and then some fat), until your body intervened (luckily) and forced you to eat more food... unfortunately, the body can't tell you exactly what food to eat, so you just ate lots of low fat (which equals high sugar) processed fake foods, lean cuisine type nutritionally barren processed fake meals, and horrible fast foods... yuck....

This is actually a pretty typical modern American, especially of the female variety! (Males have their own bad normal "types", but let's work with this for now- the solutions are identical!)

And, in addition, you've probably gone regularly to the Doctor, trying to be "responsible about your health", and have been prescribed various medications for, oh, high blood pressure, migraine headaches, anti- depressants, and maybe (worst of all!) a Statin drug for high cholesterol. And you probably have various skin ailments, dry or oily, perhaps acne or rosacia, and all in all you just feel BAD. You have trouble sleeping, and feel anxious much of the time.

All of this is very common, almost inevitable for the present day and manner of living and eating...

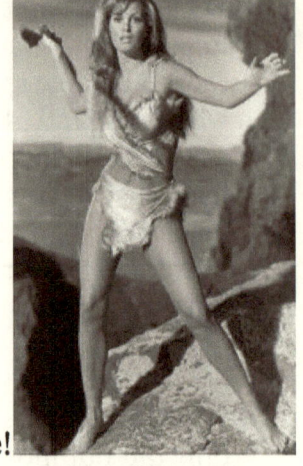

But now, let's go... Back to the Future!

Now, you are going to become the New Paleo YOU! And don't worry, it's not all that hard, in fact it's easier than what you are doing right now, and the results will amaze both you, your family and friends, and especially even your Doctor! First off, change your diet.

Actually, this is first, second, third and fourth- change the way you eat.

Simple things first- throw away your salt! No, I'm not telling you to eat less salt, I'm telling you to eat MORE! But get a good quality SEA SALT, not that lousy fake processed salt made by big industry. Himalayan is a great place to start!

Tastes amazing, and loaded with healthy minerals your body is craving

Next, throw away your vegetable oils and margarine and Crisco poisons! They have no nutrients at all, and are only helping to make you fat and sick- throw them out, don't even donate them to the homeless, they are better off with out them too. Again, I am not asking you to do without, just substitute UP- go buy real, pastured butter.

(Hey, this paleo thing isn't so hard yet, is it? It's just way tastier...)

For pastured butter, buy Kerrygold from Ireland or even better, Organic Valley pastured butter from the wondrous state of Wisconsin wherein I reside... for OIL, get olive oil, coconut oil, ghee (clarified butter) is also great and readily available. Do NOT get peanut oil (a legume), but real NUT oils like macadamia or almond oils are great. Coconut oil and pastured butter will be your go to butters, but real honest-to-God lard from grass fed beef and pastured pork or (my favorite) duck is to be prized!

So far, everything has been improvements to your life and diet (and your health!) Nothing hard so far... but now:

I want you to give up grains.

This is actually the key, the lynchpin of your health. This one thing will improve your health beyond all measure; make it possible for your to be ideal healthy lean self, bring you back to your new Paleo you, and improve everything!

And it's not that hard.

Basically, from now on resolve to only eat real food!
* * *

You can start just by going to bed early (proper sleep- 8 hours minimum is super important- just as important as what you eat, really! Get to sleep EARLY!)

And then, get up early, in time to make a good, solid, filling, make-your-body-happy-for-the-first-time-in-a-long-time breakfast!

And also in time to pack a super nutritious Paleo Lunch- a big, giant salad, with lots and lots of beef, or chicken, or tuna, or salmon, or ALL of the above would be great! Don't forget to add a lot of good quality FAT, in the form of olive oil and apple cider vinegar along with it.

Then, come home and either fire up the grill (like me!) and make a nice steak, chicken, grill some bacon for tomorrow's breakfast (and a little 'snack' for tonight too!), seafood, maybe grill a baked sweet potato to top with real sour cream and butter... not sounding too bad yet, is it???

The main thing is to stay really, really full, especially at first. Then temptations are easy to avoid...

But, I have realized over time that the very best way to implement this New Paleo You approach is with is a good Paleo Smoothie in the morning. Get a Vitamix blender, a good supply of real God-made foods, veggies, cod liver oil, coconut milk, berries, and you will have the battle already mostly won.

You have a big canister of smoothie, and if you have a glass in the morning of the most nutrient dense food on earth, trust me, your body will be utterly happy and you will not be hungry for longer than you will believe.

You will have no desire for neolithic (GRAIN) foods, devoid

of nutrition, because you have had all the nutrition you need!

This is huge. The reason modern folks are hungry virtually all the time is because they are eating things that give their bodies no nutrition- so your body says "EAT EAT EAT"!, And you do, but what you eat, again, has no nutrition!

So, the EAT signal never stops!

But now, for you, IT DOES!!

Just eat lots of real food, LOTS! To get a Vitamix to help you easily process, actually chew up the food for you and get it into your thankful body, go to paleojay.com and click on the Vitamix link. You'll get free shipping, which is the best deal on the Vitamix you will find anywhere, and also help support this wonderful show, which is the best deal you will get on a show anywhere (free)!

Oh, and after the first day, what do you do? REPEAT!

That's right, day after day, you just eat the healthiest foods on the planet (and any other planet as well!)-

Nutrient density is the name of the game! Meats, grass fed is best, pastured pork is best, free range chicken is best- bacon, steaks, pork chops, roasts, barbequed chicken, more bacon, shish-ke-bobs, more bacon, seafood, shrimp, scallops, sardines, mussels, tuna, salmon- you get the drift! Just really good, really real God made foods- EAT THE FATTED CALF!! This information is just loaded into and peppered throughout the Bible!

And, as for exercise? I know, you'll go crazy, thinking you need to "burn calories" and need to "feel the burn" as Jane Fonda infamously said...

But I, PaleoJay say to you, now- Do NOT exercise for 30 days!

Even I can't believe I just said that! But I mean it-

It is SO much more important that you understand and start into really DOING these dietary changes, that I want you to have NO DISTRACTIONS.
Your future health, your body composition (fat to muscle) ratio, your need for poisonous medications- all of this is based 90% PLUS on DIET alone!

And this from someone who does some exercise just about every single day...

But, at this point, exercise is not what you need, my friend. You need a...

New Paleo You! And you will get it- let's go back to the future!

Start tomorrow! Keep me posted on your progress. This first week is 100% about diet, and diet alone! KEEP ME POSTED!

I have a Speak pipe feature on my site,www.paleojay.com, where you can just talk into your computer to ask me a question, or even tell me that I'm a creep if you want...

Go ahead and use it son (or daughter!)...

And take some before pictures for yourself, because in about 90 days, your after pictures will be amazing!

Why a Paleo Green Smoothie?

A VITAMIX IS A CHEWING MACHINE

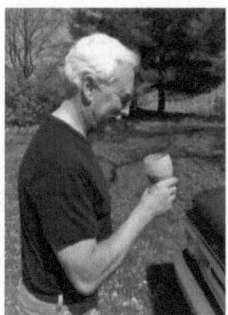

OK- here I am with a Green Drink from my Vitamix- Paleo Smoothie! I would be hard-pressed to eat this many vegetables in a day, much less chew them enough to ensure adequate digestion! With a Vitamix doing the "chewing" for me, this is not a problem!

Lots of us are not that enamored of eating lots and lots of vegetables... understandable! But, just add them to the Vitamix canister, along with some natural berries and other fruits, coconut milk, and- well, the complete recipe is in the very next chapter.

And variations are not only acceptable, but encouraged. More veggies- more variety- more health! Your garden (or your Farmer's Market!) is your Palette- draw from it- add to your health.

I know from experience that most folks resist buying a Vitamix:
1. Too expensive
2. Too big of a change of lifestyle (versus pouring

cereal and milk into a bowl...)

    3.   Seems "weird"- putting veggies and "strange" liquids (kefir, raw eggs, pastured butter, coconut milk, green tea) into a blender....

Trust me, have you priced a diagnosis of cancer or diabetes lately?

WAY more than a Vitamix.

If things in our health care system made sense, then our health insurance would cover a Vitamix, cod liver oil, perfect pushup devices, pull-up bars, and such like...but our health care system makes no sense whatsoever, which is why it (and we) are going broke! But you don't have to go down this self-destructive path-

Take the conservative approach- don't rely on Government! Provide for your own health!

Eat good, real, natural, God-made foods!

Do natural, non-machine, real body exercise!!

SLEEP a LOT!

Have good personal connections- a "Tribe" or "Family" with which you connect...

Do all of the above, and you will be a healthy, happy, spiritually fulfilled, and FIT cave person.

#

THE PALEO GREEN SMOOTHIE MASTER RECIPE!

And so, you have here revealed to you the Rosetta Stone of easy Paleo-style nutrition-
JUST ADD A VITAMIX!

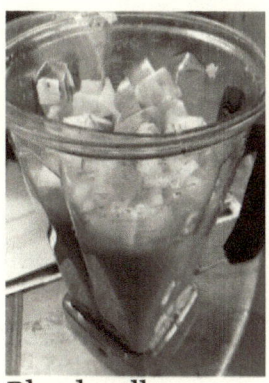

Blend well...

About a cup of green or white tea
Coconut Milk- 1 can
Carlson's or Nordic Naturals Cod liver oil- 1 Tablespoon
Powdered kelp- 1 teaspoon
turmeric powder 1 tsp
ginger powder 1 tsp powder or small section of ginger root
kelp powder 1 tsp
spirulina powder1 tsp
Maca powder 1 tsp
cinnamon- 1 tsp- also great on coffee and whipped cream!
Fresh ground is best-
These are strong anti-inflammatory agents, among many other benefits.
4 Tablespoons Bob's Potato Starch! This is key for feeding your gut microbes!!
Vitamin D3 liquid- a few drops
Unsweetened kefir- 1/4 cup
Organic, unsweetened lemon juice- 3 teaspoons OR 1 peeled lemon

PaleoJay's Smoothie Cafe!

Apple cider vinegar- 1 Tablespoon

Frozen spinach or kale or other leafy green- approximately 1 cup

Frozen mixed "California Mix" vegetables (broccoli, cauliflower, carrots), ~1 cup

Frozen mixed berries- blueberries, raspberries, strawberries- 1 cup

1/2 banana (I freeze mine so they don't over-ripen)-optional

1 peeled orange

1 peeled lemon

2 raw, organic free range eggs (optional) or more! I often use 4 eggs; the yolks are the best part, nutritionally speaking! Who needs fake protein powders?

Greek yogurt is also a good protein source, and like Kefir has lots of good gut microbes!

I know that, at first glance, the above routine seems like a LOT! But, if you set things up once, in an orderly manner, it goes really quickly- my smoothie, which I make once every 3 or 4 days usually, takes about 10 minutes, start to finish. Here are some tips:

Get some spice jars, in fact if you buy the turmeric, ginger, kelp, mac, and spirulina powders IN little spice jars, with shaker lids, you are SET. All you need to do is line them up on your counter or in a low cupboard like I have, and just go down the line when making your smoothie, shaking some of each
jar into your Vitamix canister- quick and easy!

You'll notice I start with the canister on the counter by the spices, tea and coconut milk can- then, I move over to the refrigerator and pull out those items, and then the freezer if I am using the frozen foods... by the way, fresh is just as good as frozen, and when I have my garden and farmer's market produce available I use that instead!

Then, I move over by the sink, and add in the orange and lemon there where I can peel them, and save the peelings into the compost container I keep handy.

In other words, you come up with a system, and the smoothie making becomes effortless!

The last tip I would give you, is this: after you pour off a wonderful glass of your Smoothie from the canister, take the rest of the drink and divide it into Ball canning jars- you know the kind, with the interchangeable lids! Store these in the fridge, and you are set for several days worth of health!

Quite frankly- if you start making a daily smoothie similar to the above daily, you will be doing more to improve and salvage your health than anything else I can think of! We are all suffering from years of substandard nutrition, since we are all suffering from many years of misinformation and propagandizing about long, slow exercise and low-fat nutritional lies. We have to be pro-active in rebuilding our sadly lacking health through adding in all the nutrient density we can.

This Smoothie will do that- restore your health- give you glowing skin, healthy, vital teeth and hair, and a restored immune system from the "inside out", as the beneficial bacteria are restored in your intestinal tract that digest many foods for you.

To complete your nutritional rebirth, after starting in with the above, get going with a Weber Grill, making a cornucopia of foods weekly that will last you through the week!

Just reheat later, and you'll easily have a week's worth of lunches and dinners after an enjoyable "grill outing" in your yard on a Sunday afternoon!

* * *

37

The other thing I would recommend?

Get a crock pot!
You can throw together a great Paleolithic meal in the morning, just after you make your Paleo smoothie, and before you do your Paleo Exercises!

Trust me, after you get into it, this early morning stuff will become the highlight of your day- especially the EXERCISE!

Don't know what to make in a crock pot?
Go to www.civilized caveman crockpot recipes
Now you do!!

This stuff really is not all that hard! It just requires... change... but this change is so worth it!

It means health, and vitality, and mental health (our crappy modern diet is just as bad for our mental health as our physical health)!

I think that you are worth the effort to do this, my friend! Now, just do it, for the sake of you and yours!

#

DON'T **FATTEN** YOURSELF LIKE A FARM ANIMAL!

It's already happened to us all: we all have been ingesting antibiotics for years! Primarily through medicines given us rightly, or wrongly and unnecessarily through medical doctors prescriptions since we were young, but also by eating animals that have been fed loads of it.

In the 1950's, a new drug was developed- the first antibiotic, something that would kill microbes! At the same time, it was discovered that this same drug, this antibiotic, would make animals gain substantial amounts of weight! Of course, this sounded great to farmers and ranchers, who are paid for the animals by the pound, and so they jumped on board.

They bought low grade, leftover antibiotic "slurry" from the manufacturing process by the tank load, and watched their cattle and chickens grow really fat, really fast.

And another thing: they noticed that the animals that were fed this antibiotic laced feed also seemed to not get infections easily, at least for the short life that they led up until their slaughter.

And so, the Confined Animal Feeding Operation or CAFO was born- animals could now survive in filthy, overcrowded conditions better, thanks to antibiotics!

In fact, in 1955 Pfizer sponsored a contest among pharmaceutical salesmen to see who could gain the most weight. (1955 was very different from today- it was a time when bigger was better, even in people!)

The salesmen who took antibiotics gained much more weight than those who did not.

The other thing that was happening, though, is that although the antibiotics were truly wonder drugs in healing bacterial infections, they were literally "carpet bombing" anyone who took them, destroying beneficial bacteria in the patients system that did helpful things like, oh, regulating weight and appetite, digesting and then releasing helpful compounds from foods that helped our mood, cognitive abilities, and many other facets of our lives.

And now, about 1/3 of Americans are obese, and about 5%

are severely obese.

We weigh on average 25 pounds more than we did in the 1960's, and children are much fatter and are even coming down with adult onset or type 2 diabetes in grade school!

So, if you want to "lean out" and go back to the 1950's: Only take antibiotics if you really need them for an acute infection. Look at it as seriously as surgery!

Try to avoid CAFO animals, and go for local, pastured chicken and beef and pork.

Build your beneficial gut microbe health by eating probiotics like real fermented sauerkraut and pickles, kimchi and kefir. Consider taking soil based probiotics, but definitely get out gardening, and walking barefoot, and otherwise getting in touch with the soil- good soil is absolutely loaded with the microbes we evolved with, and are as much a part of us as gravity. Without them we perish!

Feed your gut microbes by eating resistant starch! This means undigestible parts of starchy plants like really green bananas and plantains, raw potato, and potato starch in an unheated form. Ideally, this means including these foods in a Paleo Smoothie made in your trusty Vitamix on a daily, or near daily basis!

Keep the "Prebiotics for BAD bacteria" out of your system- this means keep out sugar, all forms of bread and pasta (which immediately turn INTO sugar) and all other forms of gluten, which is a harmful component of wheat. Sugar feeds the bad bacteria that infects us, and makes us sick. Also, skimmed milk is another form of sugar to be avoided at all costs- heavy cream is actually good for you though!

* * *

PaleoJay's Smoothie Cafe!

That's about it. If you do all of that- avoid sugar and grains, eat lots of healthy, pastured and wild caught animals, and plenty of fat from pastured animals, fatty fish like salmon and sardines, along with your daily Paleo Smoothie loaded with pastured eggs, pastured butter, coconut oil and milk, and loads of veggies and some berries, both you, and your gut microbes will be
in healthy and happy synergy.

I feel it in my gut!

What NOT to eat and drink!

CURE YOURSELF OF HEADACHES AND MIGRAINES

* * *

Even if you have suffered from chronic headaches and even migraines for years, it is quite possible to eliminate them, or at the very least minimize them in a completely natural manner. The key point is to adopt a paleo or ancestral type of diet, eliminating gluten entirely, and sugar as much as possible. This is the perfect first step, and hopefully you have already done
it... if not, this is, as I said the first step.

Primary suspect in this case- GLUTEN! Bread, pasta, wraps, pizza, donuts, in other words primarily wheat products- your body really doesn't need them at all, and ever since wheat was genetically altered in the 1960's and it's gluten content, particularly certain harmful elements were magnified exponentially. These components of modern wheat gluten are harmful in many ways, including destroying the intestinal vili, and harming the microbes in the gut biome.

 Just think of it this way: eating modern wheat products is like pouring acid into your gut lining!

Ironically, ancient versions of wheat, such as Einkorn wheat which is wheat from biblical times, seem to be relatively harmless to the gut, and to our health. But, given what we've just learned, that makes perfect sense, doesn't it?

So, let's say we've eliminated gluten- we have sandwiches made with lettuce wraps instead of modern wheat bread, and otherwise just eat meat, vegetables, a few starches like white rice or ancient grains, and maybe a sweet potato or baked white potato on occasion, along with lots and lots of green vegetables!

#

CUT THE GOVERNMENT GLUTEN- BUT EMBRACE REAL NUTRIENTS

The big thing now, nutritionally, is to go "gluten free", and believe me, that is a fad that is worth following! Gluten, from wheat primarily in the American Standard American Diet aka S.A.D. is a protein found in wheat that is extremely caustic and damaging over time to the intestines of mammals. It was increased greatly in the 1970's in what was called at the time "The Green Revolution", when wheat was altered to increase yields.

And it did increase yields, big time! Unfortunately, nobody thought to test things like increased "anti-nutrients" like gluten and gliadin in this new wheat- they just looked at the yields, and went ahead full bore, replacing the wheats of the bible and before like Spelt and Einkorn that waved majestically 6 feet or more in the air, and replaced them with squat, gluten loaded monstrosities that yielded many more grains per acre, but at an as-of- then undetermined cost in side effects. And so, yes, please, give up gluten!

But this is not the end of the story, and to simply replace all of our beloved processed foods and junk food with those made without gluten is an improvement, but rather slight when compared to gaining real health! Along with eliminating wheat, we need to start adding in all of the nutrients that wheat has replaced over the years- cut the wheat, but vastly increase the green veggies, the cultured full fat dairy (preferably raw), the organ meats, and the FAT!

This is probably the hardest concept to get across to people who have never really experienced the benefits of an

44

ancestral or paleo type of diet. After being brainwashed for over 50 years to cut the fat- eat low fat this and that, and skimmed milk, and margarine instead of butter- it is hard for folks to fathom that yes, indeed, their grandparents had been right, and modern medical advice has been dead wrong for at least 50 years.

The truth? Orange juice is bad- it's just sugar water- ditto all fruit juices. And sugar is worse for you than smoking cigarettes- really! It is the most cancer stimulating substance known- also, it will cut your insulin sensitivity, setting you up for diabesity, which is just the first stage of diabetes, obesity, progressive heart disease, cancer and alzheimer's and many other auto-immune diseases.

They all get started in your "leaky gut", which begins with wheat and sugar, continues with the ravages of industrial seed oils like soy and corn and canola and peanut, margarine and other nutrient lacking oils...

Take charge- cut gluten, then add in lots of fat- pastured butter, free range eggs, lots of wild caught seafood (sardines are great) cod liver oil, and everything I recommend you put into your daily Paleo Green Smoothie!

This fulfills the package, and lets your body truly rebuild and thrive from the inside out, repairing all the damage that has been done eating the "low fat LIE" diet over the years.

Cook for yourself and your family, go back to the days when we provided our nutrition for ourselves using real God made foods from nature, and turn your back on man made, processed foods promoted by Big Government and Big Corporations through subsidies provided by your tax dollars...

* * *

45

Throw out the Government Gluten, but at the same time embrace Real Foods with Natural Nutrients!

#

VEGETABLE OILS LIKE MARGARINE SUCK!

One concept that many people on the paleo journey kind of don't really get is why you shouldn't consume vegetable oils.I mean, it's just a little oil, and it comes from plants, like peanuts and corn and soy and canola, so what's the big deal?

It's a vegetable after all, right?

Wrong. Vegetable oils like canola (which is actually made from the rape seed plant and renamed for marketing purposes in Canada where most of it is grown) are highly refined, industrial seed oils. You can easily find videos on youTube that show how it is made- these videos are usually supposed to be extolling the virtues of the oil, but just look at the process as it is portrayed- the heavy machinery needed to extract oil from a hard seeded plant like rape seed or corn, the extreme heating and hydrogenation and harsh chemical extraction...

After witnessing just how vegetable oils are made, almost like refining gasoline, you will wonder why anyone could deem such fake foods even faintly edible!

Because they are loaded with trans fats, which means they are modified to be solid at room temperature, vegetable oils and especially margarine are especially harmful to your heart health. Soy and Canola oils are especially loaded with trans fats, and so are incredibly harmful- avoid them both!

Another problem with vegetable oils is that they are completely Omega 6 fats, which is a real problem in the S.A.D. standard American diet. Our diet is completely

46

flooded with this Omega 6 oil, which should be equally balanced with Omega 3 oils, which is what you get from butter, olive oil, seafood, and pastured meats.

If these two types of oil ratios get out of whack, extreme inflammation results throughout the body. Inflammation like this is what causes virtually all modern disease, and so should be avoided at all cost. Getting rid of vegetable oils and replacing them with heart healthy butter and coconut oil will go a long way towards getting rid of inflammation in the body, and also keep you satiated after meals (real fat is very satiating!) so you will stay both healthy AND slim!

There are many other problems with vegetable oils:

In one study, increased Omega-6 in breast milk was associated with asthma and eczema in young children

Studies in both animals and humans have linked increased Omega-6 intake to cancer

One study shows a very strong correlation between vegetable oil consumption and homicide rates

The Omega-6:Omega-3 ratio in blood has been found to be strongly associated with the risk of severe depression

In addition, it has been shown that the trans fats in vegetable oils are very alien, since they are not natural to the human body (we never ate them until about 100 years ago). But the body digests them, and then can't get rid of them easily, so it stores them as body fat.

But this type of strange fat is "unstable", trans fats can easily be altered by stimulus, for instance if the trans fat was stored in the skin after digestion, it could easily alter upon exposure

47

to sunlight and become a melanoma, the deadliest form of skin cancer!

And if it was stored as body tissue in the arteries, it could easily alter in a manner that promotes clotting, which could result in a heart attack.

I hope I've convinced you of the incredible evils of vegetable oils, which are better termed industrial seed oils. And bottom line- why deny yourself healthy, satisfying, totally natural God made fats like butter, cream, lard, coconut oil, and even fish oils?

Cod liver oil is one of the best foods ever- try to have some every day! If you make a Paleo Green Smoothie like I recommend, that should be one of the ingredients, and after you make it in your blender you can store several days worth of smoothie in Ball canning jars in the fridge, and you will be a nutritional golden child.

So do it- get started! Throw out your vegetable oils and margarine, buy good pastured butter (Kerry Gold or Organic Valley), a big jar of coconut oil (get two- one for the bathroom- best moisturizer ever!) and one for the kitchen.

So go ahead, and become the healthiest, happiest you that you can be- it all starts with nutrition!

#

YOUR WATER IS SLOWLY POISONING YOU

Here is the thing- your water is probably poisoning you, slowly but surely!

Unless you have a good source of well water on your property, that is free from farm fields runoffs of pesticides

48

and chemical fertilizers, you are dependent upon city water.

This is water that your city or town has come up with a plan
to treat, whether it comes from a municipal well or from a
large, polluted lake (like in Chicago!).

And when I mean "treat" your water, I mean that they dose it
with chorine, fluoride, and the recently added Chloramines,
which are a combination of chlorine and ammonia.
Chloramines, now being added to nearly all municipal water,
are so strong that they can dissolve your very pipes and
fixtures, and release heavy metals into your water. Lots of
problems here!

Fluoride is particularly troublesome, and something I really
hate being purposefully put INTO our water supply! It is
supposed to prevent tooth decay, but like the flu shot, and
the low fat high carb diet, there is absolutely NO
SCIENTIFIC BACKING TO THESE CLAIMS!

And the downside is really bad. It can effect your thyroid,
cause "fluorosis", which is an unsightly discoloration on your
teeth, affect your bones as well, and make you more prone to
cancers, dementia, bone fractures and arthritis.

Believe me, this is only the tip of the iceberg here... ONLY the
USA puts this poison fluoride purposcly into thcir watcr, of
all developed countries! It really has no positive effect on
dental health, despite the hype.

  Now, if you are like me, this makes you physically sick to
hear this stuff, and you want pure water! Understandable.

The most important thing to get, though, is not a drinking
water filter, it is a shower filter. I know, sounds
counterintuitive, doesn't it? But it is true: Chlorine is a very

strong disinfectant, and so can cause a lot of toxic issues for humans. Like an increased risk of kidney, rectal, and bladder cancers!

Asthma, and a general weakening of the immune system are other high risks of chlorine exposure.

Ironically, breathing in this chlorine, while bathing or showering, is dramatically worse than drinking it! So, for a "most bang for your buck" type of approach, get a shower filter that filters out this chlorine. Vitamin C works well for reducing chlorine, and so a Vitamin C shower filter is a great option. I

In addition, this type of filter also removes chloramines, which are even more damaging to your health! There are also some excellent whole house chlorine filters, but these start at around $1500 or so.

Best bang for the buck is definitely a Vitamin C shower filter- you can pick one up on Amazon for around $60. You can also get refills of Vitamin C in replaceable canisters, and then you will really be protecting the health of yourself and your family!

Personally, I have well water, and so have a reliable source of pure, untainted water. But if you rely on city water, get yourself a filter!

And to neutralize fluoride in the water that you drink, get yourself a Berkey type of carbon block filter. This type of filter is so powerful that it can purify water from any random stream, and make it pure and chemical, sediment, and bacteria free! A great health, and a great preparedness tool.

#

Don't eat Industrial Seed Oils Dude!

This is a key point of paleo health that is often sidelined. I mean, we all know that avoiding grains is key, but what is so bad about some clear looking oil that is labeled "heart-healthy" by every doctor and government health agency?

Well, first of all, almost every doctor and government agency is not your friend- they have an agenda; the doctor is an agent of large medical establishments that want your (and your insurance companies) MONEY, first and foremost. Besides, they have been trained by pharmaceutical company funded college programs, and all they know is drugs and surgeries- they know next to nothing about nutrition, unless they taught it to themselves. (Most pooh pooh nutrition altogether)

And the Government Agencies? They also have an agenda, and it is not to help you, the taxpayer...

They want to sell farm products, America's biggest export, and your health is probably better for them if you are NOT healthy! The less social security payouts they have to make, the better. They don't want a lot of old seniors around, sucking up money that they (the government) could spend so much better than you can!) Ha Ha.

Back to vegetable oils. Corn, soy, cottonseed, sunflower, and safflower oils are very high in omega-6 polyunsaturated fatty acids, which cause oxidative damage and inflammation, which dramatically raise the risk of heart disease!

It is very important to avoid these fake, industrial, unnatural fats!!

Unfortunately, almost anything that you buy in a supermarket that is packaged uses these cheap, industrial oils. And, if you go to almost any mainstream restaurant, these vegetable oils are what they use.

If you normally eat at home, and use real, natural, God made fats like butter, animal fats like lard, and coconut oil, you are building your health daily, particularly your heart health! Despite what we've been lied to about for decades, natural, saturated fat is incredibly healthy!

But if you eat out in restaurants, know that they almost ALL use bad, industrial seed or vegetable oils. And so, it is important to eat out only occasionally, since these oils are really bad on a regular basis! Even if you always order "paleo friendly" meals like meats and veggies, they will be cooked in bad oils.

Salads are great, but if you get them at a restaurant: the dressings are almost certainly industrial seed oils. It's kind of sickening, really; back in the 1950's and 60's, everything was cooked in natural lard or coconut oil, maybe butter.

I think that is why the WW2 generation is so long lived, they had really good food for the first half of their lives! (My own father, Phil, is still going strong, living at home with my mother Carolyn, and he is 95!)

Then, after Ancel Keyes and the stupid Mc Govern commission decided that fat was the villain; well, our national health has been on a huge tailspin since then. So, ignore them and eat real fat.

Try to avoid fake, industrial vegetable oils as much as possible- eat at home most of the time, and eat real food (and real fat). If you go out to eat, and they offer sauces like hollandaise or others, pass. They are undoubtedly soy oil based!

Just remember that these oils, although they kind of go "under the radar" since they are largely invisible, are really important. Bad, vegetable seed oils are like water in the gas tank, or a nail in the tire to the paleo diet- small things that seem beneath notice, but they are truly devastating to your health!

If you want a truly good oil, then just get a big bottle of cod liver oil, and put it in your daily Paleo Green Smoothie! Now that is an oil I can swear by!!

What you SHOULD eat and drink!

EAT REAL FERMENTED VEGGIES AND THRIVE
Eat Real Fermented Vegetables and THRIVE

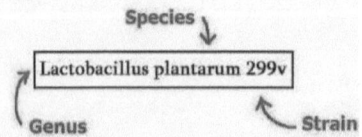

I have been an advocate of fermented veggies for a long time, but recently I have come to realize that they are very, very important indeed for your overall health!
I mean right up there with eliminating grain and sugar from your diet important...
For a long time I have repeated over and over "Add in Kefir or Greek Yogurt with active cultures into your daily Paleo Smoothie!" And this is, and was wonderful advice indeed.
But I have been reading scholarly articles (so you don't have to) and the latest rage in Paleodom is: Lactobacillus Plantarum, OR L.plantarum 299v

Hi! I'm your gut buddy!!

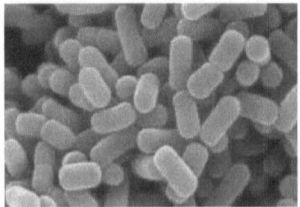

This is the fermented microbe, or "gut buddy" that lives in us all, and does really good things for us, health-wise! Perhaps most importantly, this particular, plant-based microbe protects and heals our almost always damaged intestinal linings. This means things like Chron's disease, irritable bowel syndrome, diverticulitis, anything in the gut- Lactobacillus Plantarum is what we need- it is the answer to our problem!

I had always thought that a good gut microbe was a good gut microbe... and that's true- but the rest of the story is that we need both- MILK based gut buddies- Lactobacillus acidophilus... Hence the kefir in the Paleo Green smoothie! Also, apple cider vinegar is loaded with good gut buddies, and that should be in your daily smoothie as well! But, we also need:
PLANT based gut buddies!!
Lactobacillus Plantarum, OR L.plantarum 299v!
I have long advocated that you use Kefir, or Greek yogurt to promote the Dairy based microbes of health- but NOW I know that you need BOTH varieties: SO, you need Plant based gut buddies, yes indeed you do DAILY!
But, not in your Paleo Smoothie.
Eat a pickle or two. Have some sauerkraut with your brat, or with your eggs, or your pork chop. Have some kimchi with whatever you like! Maybe on your salad...

BUT THESE ARE IMPORTANT! OUR ANCESTORS ATE THIS STUFF EVERY SINGLE DAY OF THEIR LIVES (before refrigeration), since fermentation was the only preservation available- and we have adapted to that! We NEED fermented veggies to be truly healthy! Processed foods (once again!) are found... SADLY LACKING!
So, where do you get this superfood, this wondrous health producing wonder of the Paleo era??

Ideally, you make your own- it's not hard, and kind of fun.

I'll include a link to Mercola.com that explains how to do it on a larger scale...http://articles.mercola.com/sites/articles/archive/2013/06/01/fermented-vegetables.aspx

But if you are just getting started, you might want to just BUY some fermented veggies to get started! I think this is a natural reaction, and I can relate.
Go to your local supermarket, and buy...http://bubbies.com/story
This is the only national manufacturer of fermented vegetables like pickles and sauerkraut that does it right!
 NOT pasteurized (that would kill all the gut buddies!), not just packed in vinegar to give a sour taste without any fermentation at all- their stuff is the real deal!

Farmer's Markets often have vendors that make their own fermented veggies for sale- this is also a wonderful option, just like making it yourself. But, if not available- do NOT but the mass manufactured pickles and sauerkraut and other FAKE fermented vegetables- THEY ARE NOT FERMENTED, REALLY, AT ALL!!

Don't buy them- but, if you have Asian stores in your area, pick up a bottle of kimchi! Wonderful, pungent but VERY healthy stuff!! The Asian stuff is wonderful, but the standard fermented sauerkraut and pickles are....
Just another indication of the sad state of America's food supply- things listed as healthy and wholesome are usually... NOT! Caveat Emptor- "Buyer Beware"!

As true today as it was in Imperial Rome, which we are coming to resemble more and more each day! High taxes, destruction of the small land holders in favor of the rich, politically connected BIG land holders, profits over quality, money over health...
The list goes on and on.

* * *

Back in the latter days of Rome, those with her original values moved "back to the land"... FAR from Rome- out to Spain, and France, and even Britain! They decided to provide for themselves, as much as they could, since the Empire itself was rotten and decaying.

I am sad to say, but we are in a similar situation today. REMOVE yourself, as much as possible, from BIG government. Ignore their recommendations. Do what YOU know to do be best:

1. Eat real, God made food- not processed crap
2. Avoid grains and sugars, that are in all the sterile foods recommended by the Government via the FDA and the Food Plate
3. Rely and trust your local neighbors and friends, NOT the BIG Government bureaucrats
4. Use your God given common sense- do what your grandparents would have done, about EVERYTHING- physically, mentally, spiritually- to quote the Wizard of Oz
5. Eat fermented foods

Buy a Vitamix! Best way to eat real foods in the modern world!

\#

MICROWAVING YOUR FOOD IS GOOD

I'm sure that many of you have read articles about the evils of microwaved foods...

* * *

PaleoJay's Smoothie Cafe!

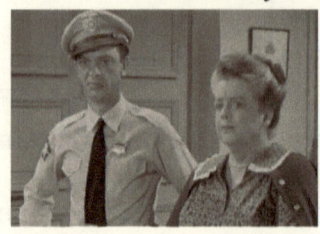

I know I have, and so I endeavored to come to the bottom of the issue. And the bottom is- (drumroll)-
Microwaving your food and beverages is not only SAFE-
It preserves nutrient value BETTER than most other forms of cooking!
So there.

I think the main problem is that we ALL, me included, have an innate distrust of what we perceive as processed foods. And rightfully so! Industrially processed and FAST foods are indeed largely unhealthy, and pernicious not only in how they affect our health, but also in how they effect our home lives by supplanting family meals, meal preparation, and just a wholesome life centered around the home and the kitchen.
BUT, and this is important, sometimes we need to look at the whole picture:
Sure, Aunt Bea didn't use a microwave, since it was not yet invented!

BUT, she WOULD have, and not skipped a beat in Mayberry, since it would simply have been another invention that would have made her daily meal preparation so much easier and efficient- for instance, if there had been one in the courthouse, Andy and Barney could have heated their meals there- Aunt Bea wouldn't need to bring them down from the house...

Mayberry aside, we don't want to be Paleo LUDDITES-

people who fear technology, and shun it as entirely EVIL. All technology is not necessarily evil at all, and microwaving our food, and iPhones, and computers, all seem to fall into this camp of USEFUL TECHNOLOGY.

Such technology should be prized, not feared!

If you're not convinced yet, well then go ahead and give up microwaves! It won't hurt you to do so...

But it sure won't help you, or your health, at ALL.

#

RAW DAIRY- A PERFECT FOOD!

"And the Lord said, I am come down to deliver my people out of the hand of the Egyptians and unto a good land, a land flowing with milk and honey."

Did you know that the forerunner to today's Mayo clinic, the Mayo foundation was place where the principle treatment was using raw milk as a cure for many diseases? It's true- in 1929, the founder of Mayo, J.E. Crewe, M.D., wrote a book entitled Raw Milk Cures Many Diseases.

Here is an excerpt: *"For fifteen years the writer has employed the certified milk treatment in various diseases and during the past ten he had a small sanitarium devoted principally to this treatment. The results obtained in various types of disease have been so uniformly excellent that one's conception of disease and its alleviation is necessarily changed."*

It has been substantially proved through many, many studies over many decades that the nutrient composition of raw milk from healthy cows, raised in sanitary conditions on good feed, is vastly superior to commercial, pasteurized milk. The only reason big agribusiness milk requires pasteurization is

59

because these cows are generally not raised in sanitary conditions, but are instead crowded together inside, in filthy conditions, to get "the most milk for the buck!"

And the "milk" from these cows is not even vaguely in the same class as the real milk that most of us still cannot even buy, since in many states it is illegal. Can you imagine: here in Wisconsin, "America's Dairyland" (it's right on our license plates!) it is **illegal** to buy raw, real milk from your neighborhood farmer! You are supposed to consume fake, sugar-water skimmed milk, ideally, because it is "low in fat". What a joke!

The fat in the milk is what carries all the nutrition which makes raw milk one of the most healthy, nutritious foods on the planet. A food that once was thought to have been consumed since 10,000 years ago, but now archeological evidence indicates that 30,000 years ago people in the High Sinai Peninsula at the north end of the Red Sea used fences to aid in confining and breeding antelope for their milk.- They likely were one of many cultures that used milk long before the beginnings of agriculture.

So now you see, raw milk has been a mainstay of health and wellness for a long, long, long time!

In fact, there is no food better for you than raw milk- now, at last, there is a bill in front of the Wisconsin legislature to legalize raw milk once again! I have called my state legislator, and I was told he would support it. But why was it ever taken away is a legitimate question.
So let me end up with a quote from Dr. Ron-

"The same repressive, reactionary forces that have concentrated power and wealth into the hands of a few have outlawed raw milk and destroyed the ability of small

*farms to survive and thrive – and ushered in the epidemic
of heart disease, cancer and other chronic problems
plaguing the modern world.*
*Raw milk is the key to the health crisis, the farm crisis, the
economic crisis, the small town crisis, even the
environmental crisis, the political crisis and the educational
crisis. Farmers who could freely advertise and sell raw milk
and its products, and fresh quality meats, free of
government intervention and hassles, could prosper, and
their communities could blossom. The restoration of our
individual and national health could become reality."*

Amen to that!

#

SKIP BREAKFAST TO BURN FAT

What do you eat for breakfast? Please go to
www.paleojay.com and leave a comment- I really want to
know what are common breakfast choices among you all.

A really great breakfast choice is a Paleo Smoothie! But
today, I'm here to tell you about Skipping breakfast! I know-
it's the most important meal of the day and all that....and,
most days, I have a big glass of my Paleo Smoothie, chock-
full of all sorts of vegetables, some berries, a peeled orange or
two, kefir, green tea... the list goes on and on- a veritable
powerhouse of nutrition! I also have eggs, sometimes bacon
and or grass fed beef sausage, perhaps some greek yogurt
with some raspberries mixed in. But, this is because on
MOST days, I work out in the early morning, about 5:30
AM. AFTER a workout is when your body is READY to
rebuild, and can actually use insulin in a GOOD way, by
pushing sugars and carbs to rebuild and expand your muscle
tissue, instead of shunting these materials into FAT.

Especially if your body has become accustomed to a lowish carb diet, say 30 to 50 grams per day for a week or so- then, on ONE day, (mine is almost always Sunday)- SKIP breakfast! A number of good things will happen:

Your body will BURN FAT, since you have accustomed it to doing so already through restricting carbs throughout the week

You will NOT get hungry, since your body is happily burning its own fat for fuel, which is a very efficient fuel source, AND

A very beneficial process called AUTOPHAGY starts in your body during this brief "fast".

This is where your body starts "cleaning house"; consuming it's own damaged and pre-cancerous, and other "junk" cells, restoring a healthy balance. If you are constantly eating and digesting, the body cannot perform this process- and it is a very important process indeed! Our ancestors did NOT eat 3 , much less 5-6 meals (and snacks!) per day! They were lucky indeed to get ONE meal, and that would usually be after exercising (stalking and killing the game that made up their one meal!). This is how we are created, it is what our bodies need and want for maximum health.

At any rate, it's fine if you have a cup of coffee in the morning,(mine is usually topped with heavy whipped cream, cinnamon and cloves; sometimes with a spoonful of coconut oil melted in as well- YUM!) The longer you wait to eat, the more fat you'll burn, but don't let yourself get hungry- have a smoothie or some eggs and bacon around noon or so, but plan your workout today (on your "fasting/relaxing" Sunday) in the afternoon...

PaleoJay's Smoothie Cafe!

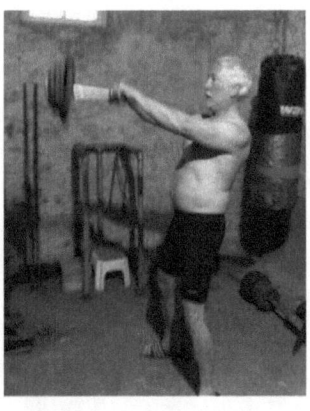

Kettle bell swings!

2 or 3 PM is about right- make this workout a TAXING one- I don't mean long, I just mean hard- Do things like negative pushups, hindu squats, chins and dips, kettle bell swings, leg raises- depending upon your ability just push pretty hard- it should be invigorating, and not so hard that you dread it-You should start to look forward to it- finish up with some barefoot sprinting if it's warm out, otherwise just do intervals of your kettle bell swings or else do intervals on a stationary bike, or even just jumping up and down! Really- that's actually a great workout move! Exercise is addressed more fully in my other eBook, Perfectly Paleo Exercise, which is also available on iTunes, Amazon and the rest- just go to www.paleojay.com, again, and all the links are right there to click on. Also, of course, right in this book as well!

Now, after your afternoon workout, is where the magic happens! You have just achieved an Intermittent Fast- a night of sleeping (not eating then, of course), and then you extended it throughout the morning. You have burnt a ton of fat, and worked out in a largely fasted state, especially low in carbs and sugars...Now, after your workout, it's time to REALLY enjoy your Sunday!

Take a shower, and then, if you're like me, fire up your grill!

Start eating good food, PARTICULARLY CARB FOODS you don't usually load up on- have a nice big early supper of meat or seafood, and also have sweet potatoes with plenty of pastured butter, white rice, or even sweet potato fries (cooked in coconut oil)- have a beer (or two!)- heck, today you can even have some ice cream or popcorn after supper! (WHAT?) Yup...
Just make sure it's all wrapped up by 6 PM or so...

When you wake up the next morning, I guarantee your waist will be visibly smaller, and your muscles will be larger and more defined (and stronger!) than they were the day before! This is called "Carb backloading", and it really does work, over and over and over again. So, just keep your carbs pretty low throughout the week, drinking a lot of super nutritious Paleo Smoothie and eating real foods as God made them naturally and not eating processed, man made junk; eat as your Great Grandparents ate, and once per week have your Fasting/Relaxing day...

You'll progress as never before, with no starving, no long hours of cardio, no depletion of energy- you'll be living in tune with your genetics, and making the inner you happy, healthy, and strong!

After doing this for a while, as I have, you will find yourself during the weeks, most nights, that you don't even feel like having supper... Congratulations- you've become a "Fat Burner"; your body prefers burning fats for fuel, and will do so most of the time!

When this happens, you will burn fat every evening and night, even if you DO eat breakfast the next morning. At this point, you have earned the right to wear a black beret and T-shirt, and hang around Paleolithic caves in France...

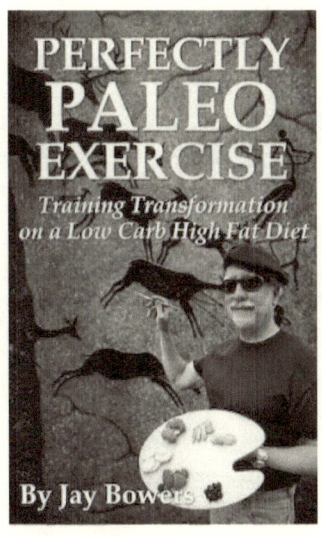

#

GRILLING OUT IS PALEO!

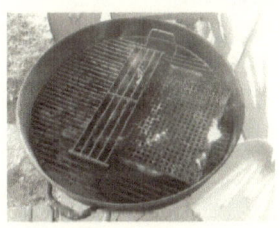

Here is my Weber grill, warming up with the Mangrate!
Also, next to the Mangrate is a PaleoJayGrate, which is just
some iron grill thing I had lying around... Just the right size
for smaller items, to keep them from "falling through" into
the fire. But I digress- the MANGRATE! I really
procrastinated on this, thinking as I do:

"Hey, this grill I inherited from my father-in-law, that is

65

from the early 1970's, works just fine. What do I need some new fangled do-dad fur... "

But, this "do-dad" is cast iron, thick and heavy- the real deal. It will leave marks on your meat, particularly steaks and chops, but actually on everything- perfectly!

I believe that grilling your meat and veggies is the most viscerally PALEO thing you can do. It literally makes you feel you are a pioneer, a barbarian, and a hunter/gatherer all in one, supplying your tribe with vittles for a long spell! Anyway, the way I do it is this:

I start the coconut shell charcoal (this is key!). This charcoal is the bomb!

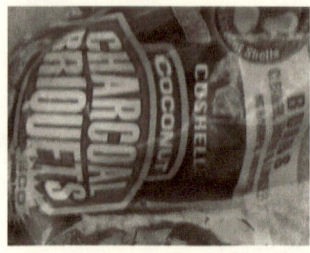

I start it with a torch!

The beauty of the torch is that, not only do you start the charcoal within about 30 seconds or so...
but you also have the opportunity at the same time to clean the grill and the mangrate!

This makes a charcoal grill actually easier (it's already superior) to a gas grill...

Just start the coals as depicted above with the torch, then put on the grill and the mangrate, and blast them with the

66

torch until clean!

Now, your coconut charcoal is glowing hot, the grill and mangrate are "flame on!", and you, my friend, are ready to grill the best food you have ever chomped!

You will probably be the new hero of your tribe!!
How good will your grilled items be? Exhibit A:

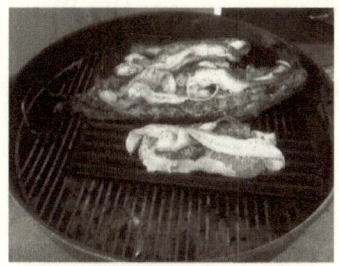

So, what have I really accomplished here? Well, the whole point is that you can easily and enjoyably spend a fun Sunday afternoon supplying your "tribe" with meat and vegetables!

You can easily prepare a week's worth of meat; just put it in your ready and waiting glass and tupperware type of containers, and you are set!

Actually, eat the meat throughout the week, and drink your Paleo Smoothie, replete with vegetables and fruits for breakfast, and all, and I mean ALL of your nutritional needs will be met.

You know, eating Paleo and enjoying life are really not all that hard, considering...
Now we have grills, Vitamix blenders, and propane torches!
(And computers and iPhones)

PaleoJay's Smoothie Cafe!

Just make sure you take the best of the old (grilling), and the best of the new (propane torches and cast iron grill grates), and ignore the worst of the new (grains and flour, sugar and processed food), and you will be golden my friend!

Like a Barbarian lurking on the outskirts of Rome, you can pick and choose what you see as valuable from "Civilization".

You can reject the decadence, you can ignore the Romish breads in favor of your own herds... but, you can adopt the Roman steel sword, and notions of sanitation and aqueducts, along with plumbing...

It is possible to have the BEST OF BOTH WORLDS!!

\#

DON'T JUST ELIMINATE BAD FOODS- ADD IN NUTRIENT DENSITY!

Let's say you've been on the ancestral, paleo, or barbarian diet template for awhile, perhaps a year or longer! You've probably improved your health and wellness quite a bit- lost fat, gained muscle, have improved digestion and health, and a new clarity in thinking. But, perhaps not....

If this is the case, perhaps you have concentrated only on eliminating bad foods loaded with anti-nutrients; things like grains, sugar, vegetable or industrial seed oils made from grains and processed, margarine- those are all wonderful things to get rid of, and doing so enables your body to begin to heal all the damage they have caused to your body and brain over the years as they were damaging your intestinal villi, and
otherwise tearing down your health.

68

But this is just Job #1!

The other half of the nutritional equation, which is every bit as important, it to add in those nutrient dense superfoods to give your body the raw materials it needs to actually BUILD excellent health!

So, just eating lots of gluten free goodies, while not as damaging as their grain-based counterparts, are still not giving your body what it needs to thrive and rebuild. You need to add in those foods that are the most nutrient dense on the planet.

If you make a green, Paleo smoothie and drink it almost every day, you are pretty much most of the way there, nutrient density-wise! I go out of my way to have it include just about everything your body needs. Think of the Smoothie as the Anti-S.A.D. diet- that diet of pizza, coke, fries, sick and abused and confined animal hamburger and chicken, noodles, fake fat, processed breakfast sugar cereals- you get the picture!

Those foods, while they are hyper-palatable, and are engineered to be that way just to sell- and they displace the foods that your body actually needs, and just give you loads of body fat and inflammation.

So, go with the Paleo Smoothie- great start! You can include the vegetable sulphur rich foods with their organosulfur compounds, and do it in a raw form very efficiently and easily, but just blending them in! Things like:

Broccoli, Cauliflower, Brussel Sprouts... These sulfurous category of vegetables have been pointed out by Dr. Terry

Wahls as a very important category of nutrient dense foods, with which idea I completely agree with her!

Terry is an important figure in the ancestral, or nutrient dense style of eating, and is coming out with a new book which I think will be a must read. Get her book, watch her viral TED talk, and absorb the information she has to offer.

Back to sulphur-rich foods: there are some other great organosulfur foods that are not really appropriate for the Paleo Green Smoothie, like:

Onions and Garlic, Shallots and Leeks

Garlic, in particular, is probably the most potent organosulfur foods you can take in! What to do? Simple- in addition to your smoothie, most days also have a giant salad- lettuce, spinach, meat or seafood, lots of real olive oil and apple cider vinegar, and lots of garlic and onions! Get yourself a good garlic press, like the ROSLE I have, and add in the anti-inflammatory, anti-carcinogenic, anti-microbial, and glutathione stimulation that this wonder food will provide- not to mention garlic tastes great!

Glutathione is particularly important, as it is the "the master anti-oxidant" that will enable your body to fight inflammation, raise energy levels, and slow down the aging process, among other wonderful properties.

Getting all of this through real foods in incredibly important.

 If you use glutathione supplements, this could shut down the production of it by your own body over time... so, just get the nutrient dense, sulphur rich foods your body needs, and let it make it's own!

* * *

Also include sulphur rich animal foods, like eggs yolks, grass fed beef liver, grass fed beef, and even high quality grass fed whey protein! (That last can go right into your Paleo Smoothie!)

And so, remember- eliminate the BAD, but also be sure to embrace the GOOD!

Sleep is MORE important than Exercise!

EARLY TO BED AND EARLY TO RISE- CRUCIAL FOR HEALTH

I've been enjoying some vacation time!

I say this not to gloat (although it has been pleasant!), but to share with you some insights I've gained over this period: Work/Activity is overrated!

All of us, Americans I believe in particular, have been brainwashed into believing that, if we are not being productive, i.e. engaged in making money, or preparing to make even more money, that we are wasting our time!

And on the other end, if we are spending our leisure time, time we have gained away from work, we had better do it productively:

Attending expensive spectator sporting events!
Luxury travel to far-distant "pre-packaged" destinations!!
Going to "spas" and "fat farms"; where we are told WHAT TO DO health wise!!!
And, don't just SIT! Watch TV!! It is at least 'mind-expanding'!!!!

I'm here to tell you, first-hand, that it is just not so!
* * *

72

Work is important; yes it's true! Crucial even- but it needs to be real work!

How many of us can honestly say today that we go to work to... labor?

To accomplish real, physical things?

Very few of us, in modern corporate America at least, can lay claim to doing so. We sit in offices, we drive to conferences, we connect and network on our computers and other devices...
We don't really do honest work anymore!

I know, I know- I am pushing the point; of course we all are "stressed" mentally and socially, and have to cope with lots of paperwork and such... but, my above point still holds.
THAT is why, when we are NOT engaged in "WORK", modern-style-

WE NEED TO REVERT TO OUR PRE-INDUSTRIAL AGE PAST!
1. Do LOTS of physical things!
Work out. Cut wood. Hike. COOK!!
2. But also other "Physical" things we ignore:
Lie around. Meditate. Ponder things. Sing and play with family and friends! Pray!!
But mainly, we need to sleep!

The last few nights, I have gone to sleep around 8 PM or so.

And then, I have slept through the night, and not gotten up until 9 AM!

This from a guy who normally wakes up and gets going at 4:30 AM!

Why? It is really a conscious decision to use my vacation to "reconnect" with my "paleo past" if you will... and I believe it really paid off!

I have had several "lucid" dreams- strongly visual dreams that are actually more meaningful upon awakening than my real, actual life! I am certain that these dreams are my "subconscious, inner self" trying to tell me what is really important.

Thinking about these dreams, and trying to interpret them, becomes more important than you would believe- if you have the leisure to actually contemplate them!

So, if you can, give yourself that leisure! If you have a vacation coming up, don't turn it into a "work substitute", where you run from event to event, just like work!

Try to actually relax; cut loose from things! If you normally work out each day, don't!

If you rarely work out- DO!

Try to eat really, really well- totally Paleo! Vacations are where we are trained to "let it all go diet-wise". Huge mistake- we want to get back in touch with our primeval selves!!

And then- sleep a lot! I mean much more than usual- try out how it was for our primeval ancestors, before electric lights and alarm clocks. Rejuvenating....

And if you don't have a vacation??

This is even more important for you:

PaleoJay's Smoothie Cafe!
* * *

Get to bed REALLY EARLY! Early enough so you will have a good 8-9 hours of sleep....

GET UP really early!! You will feel like getting up, since you've had ample sleep...

Work out, early morning! If you do this one thing, you are setting yourself up for a happy, fulfilling, and ultimately very successful day!!

Start out with "mobility-type" movements, next do some stretches- include the Asian Squat.

Follow up with self-resisted exercises, visualized resistance exercises, and isometric holds.

Finish up with pushups, sit-ups, and hindu body-weight squats.

If you do all of this, and if you are like me you will do it in front of the TV!! Netflix streaming!!

Reward yourself for working hard! You will come to LONG for your exercise sessions, if your restrict your TV watching to ONLY during those times!!

Trust me, you will feel great! Have a Paleo smoothie and toddle off to "work"-

Everything you experience there will "fall into place", and you will recognize everything for just what it really is...

And you will have some really interesting dreams to ponder, as you do your paperwork and teleconferencing and such...

#

SLEEP YOURSELF LEAN AND HEALTHY

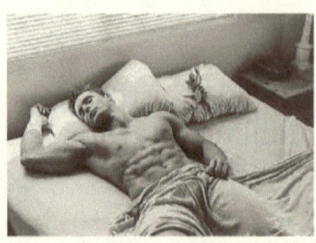

The notion of getting enough sleep seems so corny, and so simple that it can't really be that important, can it?
"I am so busy, both at work and at home, that I can't sleep more than 6 hours a night!" say most people nowadays

But if you are waking up early to work out, and then working out again after work to "burn calories" and get thinner, you are doing things very wrong...If you don't get at least 8 hours of real sleep per night, you are raising your stress hormone levels of cortisol, and increasing your chances of becoming diabetic,

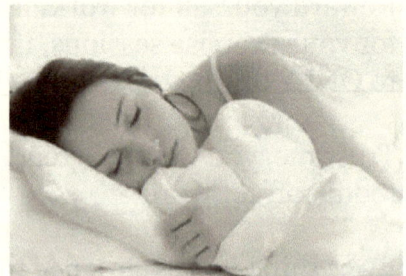

hypertensive, and obese.

Your risk of heart disease and mental disorders increase dramatically as well! So, the notion of getting a good night's sleep seems too "inconvenient", you'd better reconsider. Good, restful sleep is more important than exercise, and

76

even more important than a proper, paleo type of diet!

For one thing, if you stay up late and get up early, you will simply have more time to eat. Also, when sleep deprived, the ghrelin and leptin hormones will get out of whack, and cause an irresistible urge to eat. You cannot overcome biology.

Doesn't that sound ominous? Well, it is! So, I hope I have convinced you that late nights out or watching TV aren't "harmless" to your health goals.

So, you have become convinced, by the badgering of PaleoJay, to start getting a good 8-9 hours of sleep per night. Good for you! This will be a game-changer, a life changer really. Not only will your body become a much more efficient fat burner, your appetite will decrease, and your mood and energy level will increase. A desire for productive exercise will follow as sleep restores your mind and bodily processes. Most people don't even realize how much better they could feel on a daily basis, if they only got enough sleep!

It's like the paleo diet and lifestyle itself- once you really think about it, it is so common sense that it is undeniable:

Processed foods, loaded with sugar and artificial fats are not healthy
Altered grains, loaded with tons of gluten are toxic
Produce sprayed with toxic chemicals is not good for us
Never walking or exercising leads to a sick, debilitated and weak body
Nutrient rich foods will make a strong, healthy, lean body

Who would argue with any of these statements?? The only ones who do are those with a moneymaking agenda:

* * *

77

The Federal Government, which is in the business of selling grains, worldwide, and so has a vested interest in ignoring the health implications of consuming such a toxic foodstuff.

Big Pharmaceutical and Medicine, which is in the position of making huge profits by making us all sick (from eating these toxic grains, vegetable oil grains, processed foods (loaded with grain products like high fructose corn syrup), and other sugars.

And Big Food corporations, which make billions selling substandard, nutrient poor processed foods like breakfast cereals and snack foods made from... grains and sugars and vegetable oil crap!)

So, add one more onto the paleo, ancestral list:

8-9 hours of sleep per night is a NECESSITY!

Follow the advice of myself, and your great grandparents- Eat real food, natural God made food, exercise in nature, and get a good night's sleep each night!

"But Jay, Jay- how do I do that- get a good night's sleep I mean? I just can't sleep that long, or that soundly!"

Well, grasshopper, I have an some answers to that, and some will sound unconventional to you, but they are all true, and proven, so please do them for your own sake:

Get the television and any other electronics out of your bedroom! NEVER watch TV in bed- the bed is for sleeping, it is sacrosanct. If you have night lights, make sure they are RED, as that does not signal with the blue light spectrum that it is daytime, and you should be awake!

* * *

Download and install the https://justgetflux.com/ app onto your computer. It's a free app, and switches off the blue light spectrum gradually as it becomes later, readying you for sleep in spite of looking at your computer screen.

Black out your bedroom! If you live in an urban or suburban type of environment, you probably need blackout types of curtains. NO light should be intruding on your sleeping space!

And last, probably most important (even though you've probably never heard of it before)-

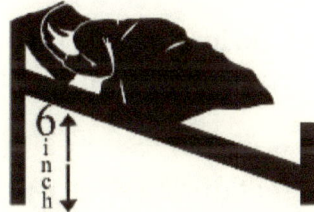

Raise the head of your bed by 4-6 inches!!

Really. This accomplishes a number of positive things, like eliminating sleep apnea, snoring, varicose veins,along with many other benefits! It does this by greatly enhancing the circulation in the body; this results in better sleep, more vivid dreams, and numerous bodily improvements which are enhanced by improved sleep.

Just put blocks of wood, or bricks, or even old books under the posts of your headboard, or get risers made to raise beds commercially, and only use them on the top end of the bed- you want the legs to be lower than the head!

The positive effects of this simple, free fix have impacted my own life dramatically- I no longer snore, I no longer have

sleep apnea, and I don't have to get up at night to use the bathroom! There are detailed scientific reasons as to why this slight elevation works, and why it is so important, but the bottom line is that it does work. If you want to explore it more, go here-
http://inclinedbedtherapy.com/

But, from my point of view, I just want you to start getting a good night's sleep! Each and every night. 8-9 hours...

Your body will start to burn fat, because it's not stressing out about the crisis it thinks you're in, since you aren't sleeping enough. In a crisis mode, your body starts to store fat!

You will start to feel great, like you do after a long vacation, where you just relax for long days, and sleep your fill day after day...

Your skin will rejuvenate (it does that during sleep), and you will start to feel and look younger, day by day.

Now, look at my watch: You are getting sleepy...

#

INCLINED BED THERAPY!

According to several researchers, traditional horizontal sleeping has been shown to prevent the ability of the body's circulatory system to function at an optimum level; thus, this sleeping position causes restricted blood flow and the inability of the lymphatic system to flush out the toxins that accumulate in the many networks of vessels throughout the body.

Inclined Bed Therapy (IBT) tends to solve this problem.

Introduced by Andrew K. Fletcher, Inclined Bed Therapy

(IBT) involves sleeping on a bed raised at the head between 4 and 8 inches using bricks, wedges or blocks. This utilizes the force of gravity to improve the circulation of the body while asleep and taking advantage of this by allowing body cells to heal and regenerate on their own. Circulation is maintained and improved from changes in all fluid densities in the lymphatic system due to gravity. For this, reports from users around the world stated that Inclined Bed Therapy can be useful in disorders such as spinal cord injury, back pain, acid reflux or GERD, sinus and respiratory disorders, sleep apnea, poor circulation, blood pressure, multiple sclerosis and diabetes.

I know, it sounds absolutely incredible! Basically the theory is that every condition of the human body, any disease or imperfection, is improved drastically by sleeping with increased circulation!

Hey, that doesn't sound so crazy, does it? Circulation is literally the lifeblood of the human body- improve that in a large way, and; well, the human body will improve from the increase in life-giving circulation.

Andrew Fletcher is the Englishman who introduced this form of therapy, after deducing that the circulation of the sap in trees is exactly like our own circulation- it is not only through the action of a "pump" (in our case, the heart), but it is the action of gravity and "transpiration", which raises the fluid in trees to hundreds of vertical feet in height.

The human body works similarly- by sleeping on a flat surface, we inhibit our circulation. The venous return of the blood is hampered by sleeping flat.

What is crazy is that sleeping with the head of the bed elevated 5-6 inches solves all of your circulation problems!

No cost, no lifestyle change- just sleep with your head elevated at a roughly 6 degree elevation!

81

PaleoJay's Smoothie Cafe!
* * *

If you have varicose veins, this is a fast, total cure. No debate; it is! But there are many, many other benefits:

Psoriasis, spinal cord injury, Parkinson's disease, cerebral palsy, bladder incontinence, bed wetting, insomnia, fidgety legs and limbs, sleep disorders, night time paralysis, multiple sclerosis, ME, CFS, diabetes, varicose veins, migraine headaches, poor eye sight, pain, bowel incontinence, acid reflux, gerd, balance problems, lethargy, poor circulation, metabolic disorders, immune deficiency, these are just some of the diseases that improve with IBT.

Ironically, standard medical practice is to elevate the foot of the bed, to make people sleep on a decline for varicose veins. This helps at first, while the patient is lying down, but as soon as he gets up the swelling comes back!

By raising the HEAD of the bed, the natural circulation is increased hugely, and in a permanent fashion. Actually, the thing to remember is this:

To lay totally flat in a bed is harder on your body than anything else you can do!

When you stand or change positions all day, or run, walk, or exercise, your circulation increases in a big way. We all know this! BUT, if you sleep in an elevated head position, your circulation during those hours is vastly improved as well. So, if you sleep like this, which is about 1/3 of your life, your health will improve by a huge, huge margin.

OK- I have done this (you knew old Paleojay would, didn't you grasshopper?), for several weeks. First, I just noticed that I slept really, really well! So did my wife, who initially was NOT on board to raise the head of the bed. But the proof was in the pudding, as they say!

Then, I looked at my feet as I exercised each morning. I have

82

veins on my feet that are kind of bright blue! Since I worked as a mailman for 38 years, and have always been a heavy exerciser, I assumed this was just extreme "foot abuse", and since there was no pain, I never really thought a lot about it... After about a week of IBT, THE VEINS HAD DISAPPEARED ON MY LEFT FOOT, AND ARE NOW HALF GONE ON MY RIGHT!

I had never even though about it- I just enjoyed sleeping really well, each and every night, and the fact that I didn't really need to get up to urinate- but then, I started to put the pieces together. All of this from just sleeping on an incline??

And here is the kicker:

NO sleep apnea. No snoring! (Just ask my wife). VASTLY improved quality of life, even though I was perfectly healthy beforehand (I thought), all just from sleeping on an incline!!??

It makes sense: the more upright you remain throughout life, the more you retain your faculties. And do you know what? In the ancient world, this was well known. Even in the Egyptian tombs of the Pharoahs, they have measured the preserved beds of these Kings...

THEY ARE ALL ELEVATED AT THE HEAD,
EXACTLY 6 INCHES!

There is even a footrest provided, so the sleeper would not slide off of the bed.

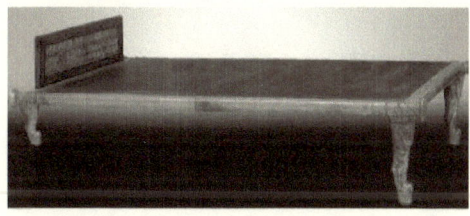

So, my takeaway point?

SLEEP LIKE AN EGYPTIAN!

PaleoJay's Smoothie Cafe!

Exercise- How much, and what kind?

EXERCISE IN YOUR MIND- VIRTUALLY!

I'll say it again, I have often enough- exercise is all about the MIND, not the exercise equipment! The more high tech, the fancier the weight lifting apparatus; generally the less it facilitates the all important mind-muscle connection.

This last is the most important thing to achieve in developing your body! Notice, I do not say how to lift the most weight- this is irrelevant. What we want to do, if you think about it, is to move your body in a manner that develops you and your body to the ultimate degree possible. NOT just "how much you can lift", all of which is determined largely by your joint and tendon attachments, and your various limb lengths relative to your torso...

What you want is to develop your own body (and mind!) to the best, natural, strong, fit and flexible, athletic and symmetrical physique you can attain- the best possible YOU!

Lifting heavy weights will not do this- you will be led to progressive and irreversible injury, with ruined joints, weak ligaments and tendons, and lifelong pain!

Running long distances won't do it- you will have ruined joints, low muscle mass, and a "skinny fat" body that at first can only run, but after a while, can't even do that!

Cross fit, Olympic lifting, power lifting, long distance

running- they all are, long term, dead ends.

I think conventional bodybuilding is also a dead end of pain, given that nowadays heavy weights are a given, but I recently heard an interview of Arnold Schwarzenegger by Tim Ferriss that was like a tonic to me. Arnold said that he eventually realized that, when he trained best, it was like a meditation. He flexed his biceps, and completely connected with his mind, flexing just by imagining lifting a weight- the weight was superfluous! By flexing, whatever muscle group he chose, and really imagining it, and making it as hard as he wanted, the stress on the muscle was ideal, and it would grow!

Virtual Resistance in action!

This is virtual resistance training, and the best first step in building your body.

Next, add in self resistance training, where one limb opposes another by pressing against it, and now you develop your tendon and ligament strength along with your muscle strength- this is key to develop raw strength and power along with the ability to sustain it without injury.

If you use heavy barbells, for instance, to build bulky, blocky muscles- these muscles will quickly outstrip the strength of their "connectors" in the tendons and ligaments, and you are setting yourself up to have your rotator cuff, and your knee joints to rupture and tear. This is no joke! Besides you winding up with heavy, saggy pecs from heavy bench presses (not a very masculine image, is it?) and a protruding abdomen and fat butt from heavy squats- you can also look forward to injured joints and torn tendons and ligaments from a misbalance between tendon and muscle relative strength.

There IS an easier, and better way!

Perfectly Paleo Exercise. I mean natural, virtual resistance exercise (ala Arnold), followed by self resisted exercise, and then body weight exercise and simple stretching, all done in your living room or in your basement or garage. Add in a once per week session using a pull up bar and/or gymnastic rings, and you will build the perfect, lifelong, functional and completely healthy and natural physique that is each of our birthrights!

And all without any injuries, expenses, commuting, or just plain PAIN that comes from things like Cross Fit or other Big Gym Box experiences. Do it yourself, at home, with your tribe, in your own cave or meadow. It's really not complicated, just like real health is not complicated- we don't need medicines, we don't need surgeries, we don't need endless drugs and procedures!!

We need good, real, God made foods like grass fed meat and dairy- real organic veggies and fruits, real fatted calf fats like- the fatted calf! Pastured dairy! Organ meats! A "tribe" to connect with- a belief in something greater than ourselves, OR ANY ONE GOVERNMENT! Land to work- a garden- a space to get our hands dirty and do REAL WORK! Not sitting in a cubicle, or driving around to meetings, or talking on the phone conferences... real work.

Our evolutionary heritage demands all of the above. There is no escape, no one else can do it for you. It's simple, and it's all do-able IN YOUR MIND.

\#

Virtual Resistance Exercise is the

PERFECT CORE EXERCISE!

This is a hard one to tackle via the written word- HOW to describe how to do a type of exercise that we all should know, and do, on a daily basis...

But that no one knows how to do anymore???

It's like how we eat in the present day- most people nowadays live almost totally on processed foods, and fast foods- in other words, "fake" foods that come in a bag or a box, require none or minimal preparation, and contain calories but almost no nutrients! We actually have forgotten how to prepare and cook our own food- this is a skill me must relearn to regain the health of our forebears, and escape the nightmare slide into diabesity, autism, autoimmune diseases, and pharmaceutical overkill for profit!

Simple things like making stock from beef bones or a chicken carcass, obtaining the nutrients from those bones which are crucial for our health- grilling meat and then eating it throughout our week, making our own soups and stews- real, healthy foods that build the health of our bodies in a huge and uber important way- foods that have been largely abandoned in modern, Government subsidized grain based diets that sabatoge our diets, destroy our health, and ensure that we are addicted to a diet that makes us very sick, and very fat, but does not kill us, as long as we take the many very expensive drugs that mask the symptoms of our many diseases, but do not effect any cure of the underlying cause.

And that is because the cure is very simple- eat real foods, mostly prepared at home, and do real exercise!!

* * *

Not joint destroying exercise like heavy weight training, or prescriptions for overtraining like P-90X or Cross fit or any of all of those overkill protocols- and no jogging/running for endless miles that only destroy your joints and muscle tissue, and produce massive amounts of cortisol, the stress hormone, that will actually encourage your body to store fat at the same time it is destroying muscle...

No- you want simple, classic, timeless, Perfectly Paleo Exercise, especially in the form of virtual resistance exercise!

But, unless you are from before the 1970's, you know nothing of Charles Atlas and his "dynamic tension", and even if you are from the 1970's and past you probably never heard of Arnold Schwarzenegger "posing" for contest prep, or of Bruce Lee and his katas and isometric holds.

All of these were expressions of the most ancient, effective, and powerful methods
of training ever discovered- Virtual Resistance Training!
This is a good modern terminology for this ultimate exercise, that requires NO equipment, can be done anywhere at any time, and builds muscle and strength without any wear and tear on the joints and tendons whatsoever-
It actually builds tendon strength as it also strengthens muscle tissue, avoiding injury from the get-go!And so- how do you do it? I will rcfcr you to my site- www.paleojay.com

Not joint destroying exercise like heavy weight training, or prescriptions for overtraining like P-90X or Cross Fit or any of all of those overkill protocols- and no jogging/running for endless miles that only destroy your joints and muscle tissue, and produce massive amounts of cortisol, the stress hormone, that will actually encourage your body to store fat at the same time it is destroying muscle...

* * *

No- you want simple, classic, timeless, Perfectly Paleo Exercise, especially in the form of virtual resistance exercise!

But, unless you are from before the 1970's, you know nothing of Charles Atlas and his "dynamic tension", and even if you are from the 1970's and past you probably never heard of Arnold Schwarzenegger "posing" for contest prep, or of Bruce Lee and his katas and isometric holds.

All of these were expressions of the most ancient, effective, and powerful methods of training ever discovered- Virtual Resistance Training!

This is a good modern terminology for this ultimate exercise, that requires NO equipment, can be done anywhere at any time, and builds muscle and strength without any wear and tear on the joints and tendons whatsoever-

It actually builds tendon strength as it also strengthens muscle tissue, avoiding injury from the get-go!And so- how do you do it? I will refer you to my site- www.paleojay.com

And also on youtube at www.youtube.com/watch? v=DI65LRENdKo- this is my easy introduction for you! Probably it would be easier to just go to youTube, and search under Basic Visualized, Perfectly Paleo Visualized Resistance Exercises !
I have several short videos of how to do these exercises there for you. You can also get my ebook Perfectly Paleo Exercise with similar videos and links. The most comprehensive example of how to do virtual resistance is at http:// transformetrics.com/exercises

John Peterson and Wendy Pett do a great job demonstrating the basics of virtual resistance training!

* * *

I know- it almost seems too simple and easy...

And it is simple- but not easy- generating the resistance
yourself is every bit as taxing and difficult as lifting weights,
and takes a LOT of mental concentration that weights do not
as much- but the results are actually superior, and will build
a far more symmetrical or beautiful type of lean, defined
physique than will weights, that build a bulky, or blocky type
of look, with a fat butt and bulging abdomen.

 And virtual resistance will also NOT build a "skinny-fat"
body, as will endless aerobics or long distance running.
Virtual Resistance exercise will build a natural, balanced,
pleasing and symmetrical physique that is like that
represented in ancient Greek statues.

A physique that is strong in real world terms of strength! A
body that has tendons that can throw, lift, twist, bend and
squat- a body ready for action, NOT for the lifting platform,
the posing dais, or any other artificial event...

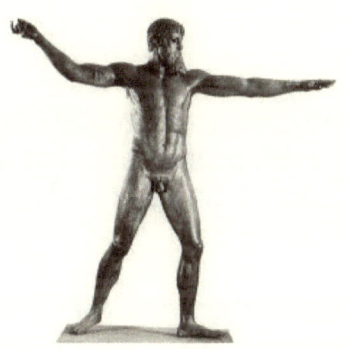

BUT A BODY BUILT FOR REAL LIFE!

#

EXERCISE EACH MORNING, EVERY MORNING

That sounds rather severe, but it really isn't- think of it as a really slow, easy way to "clear the cobwebs" and slowly rev up the old bodily and mental machinery. I don't mean to say you should bounce up out of bed and charge away to sprint, do pull ups and pushups, and then jog for an hour, followed by stretching- not at all!

I want you to slowly awaken after a full 8 hours plus of restful sleep, in a totally blacked out room. Take a series of deep, costal type breaths lying on your back in bed: inhale slowly, as deeply as you can, first expanding your diaphragm down by your belly, and then slowly filling up the upper portion of your lungs completely- then slowly exhale. Do this 5-10 times, and you will be completely awake! Go to the bathroom, and then you can go like me downstairs into the kitchen, where I start the water boiling for my coffee and tea, and do some quick warmup motions on each set of joints- elbow, neck, knees, back, shoulders- just easily rotating the joints to get the synovial fluid going, readying them for the day. Just like a CAT.

Next, I take my first cup of coffee, laced with a teaspoon or so of coconut oil, and go to the gym... my living room! Barefoot and with minimal clothing. You can do similarly, but a room with a tv or computer is really nice- there you can do your morning workout with a Netflix show on!

Spread a yoga mat on the floor, and start your exercises- for my money, virtual resistance exercises are perfect to start- they completely revitalize the body as they refresh and strengthen it. Go methodically throughout your entire musculature.

92

Then, go down to the mat and stretch! Finish with a back bridge if you can, and then go to your rebounder, and bounce on that for another 10 minutes.

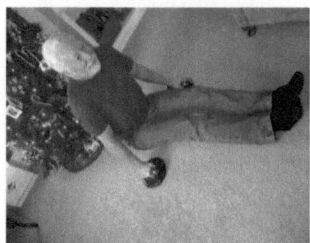

The L-Sit

Only watch your Netflix favorite while you are exercising-this will make you eager for the next morning when you can pick up where you left off. Trust me, once you've done this for awhile, you will find the perfect exercises for you, and you will relish this early morning routine. As you progress, you can add in more exercises- for instance, twice per week I also do several hundred pushups in sets of 30-40 with different hand spacings, alternating with hindu pushups, hindu squats, and straight-legged sit ups. But just twice per week maximum!

The daily routine, with the virtual resistance, self resisted exercise like curls with one limb resisting the other, the stretching and the rebounding can, and should, ideally be done daily- it is that gentle, and pleasant. But don't mistake-it is also very, very effective in strengthening every inch of your body, from your neck to your toes.

Done in this manner, daily exercise is restorative, nothing to dread but something to look forward to. And you will be setting yourself up from the start for what will inevitably be a happy and productive day!

#

BE A PHYSICAL CULTURIST- FORGET CROSSFIT,

BODYBUILDING, POWERLIFTING AND OLYMPIC LIFTING!

Back around 100 years ago and more, to be interested in health and strength and physique and just the ability to do physical things was called "physical culture". And so it remained for many, many years- and the bottom line was always, since the ancient Greeks, the cultivation of health in it's most extreme form! Since the late 1960's, this ancient ideal has been... degraded and split to the point of extremes. Today's world has as it's latest fad Cross Fit.

The idea was to reverse the split of physical culture into powerlifting, bodybuilding, and Olympic lifting and go back to ultimate fitness; I.e. What sounds like... physical culture!

But it surely has NOT turned out that way!

For one, there is FAR too much emphasis on the use of weights- not machines, but still WEIGHTS in a huge way! Cross Fit has turned into a huge competition- lift more, lift heavier, lift faster- with no end ever in sight! And have fun doing it!!

This way lies madness... it is a sure prescription for injury, overtraining and illness, and, again, extreme injury! It's expensive, cult-like, and seems to be elitist as well. I say- JUST DO IT YOURSELF!

 Do Perfectly Paleo Exercise- bodyweight exercise, self-resisted, ON YOUR OWN, and especially Virtually Resisted Exercises ala Bruce Lee, where the BODY ITSELF generates its own resistance, cat-like, within the muscle itself.

 You compete against YOURSELF only, and enjoy the

\#

PALEOLITHIC FITNESS ON THE REBOUND

As usual, I am coming to you with something that seems like it's "out of left field" somewhere- REBOUNDING! ?? Jumping on a mini-trampoline for health and fitness?

I know- at first glance, it looks like something that Richard Simmons would be promoting on late night informercials...

BUT- truth be told- rebounding is the REAL DEAL- an absolutely wonderful way to promote and enhance your fitness!

Despite the fact that it does NOT appear to be something our hunter/gatherer ancestors would have done (they wouldn't have- the technology was not available for springy jumping surfaces back then)!! - it is like many modern technologies that are VERY paleo friendly- like iPhones to look up sites like www.paleojay.com, or like the Vitamix blender that makes it so easy to liquify and thus make available all of the nutrition in leafy greens, berries, and coconut milk- (to name but a few paleo smoothie ingredients!)

What it does is to duplicate the endless, easy movement that our forebears engaged in, almost constantly- walking,

96

squatting, occasionally sprinting and jumping... and it does so in a way that is very, very safe and natural- with virtually NO stress and jarring on the ankles, feet, knees and hips as is the case with running or jogging.

You simply buy a little rebounder, or trampoline of about 3 feet or so in diameter, and put it in your living room... mine is near the television. And then, you just- bounce on it- and not necessarily hard; most of the benefits can be achieved by lightly bouncing without your feet necessarily even leaving the surface. This mild action is sufficient to not only elevate your heart rate beneficially, but more importantly it activates your lymph gland drainage system.

Most modern cubicle dwellers and car cage drivers are incredibly deficient in the simple jogging motion that our bodies have evolved to depend upon to activate our lymph, or toxin drainage system! We really need this movement to be healthy! Most folks have toxins galore welled up in their bodies, and the lymph system to cure it needs movement- preferably up and down movement- to operate!

Enter the rebounder! The iPhone of the lymph system!!

Just stand on it, and then... bounce- slightly! This alone is enough to engage the lymph system. I like to do my virtual resistance exercises while bouncing- just FLEX your muscles, as if you were a bodybuilder in a posing routine while... bouncing.
You have upped the ante- the very act of bouncing has increased the intensity of your exercise by a quantum amount.

The BALANCE afforded by rebounding is an incredible benefit, and one I believe is almost totally ignored by conventional training. Just by being on an unstable surface,

97

you are teaching your body how to balance, which is a skill quickly lost in modern, car and chair bound modern life! And, it is fun! There is something about bouncing around that brings out your inner child- kind of like barefoot sprinting! THAT surely brings out the 8 year old Jay- and so does rebounding! It is just pure PLAY.

Also, if you suffer from plantar fasciitis (as so many do today), this rebounding is akin to running barefoot in sand- it is wonderful for restoring the strength in your shoe-wearing atrophied feet. Our feet are elaborate extension bridges of tendons and muscles, as I have mentioned before: constant wearing of shoes, or "casts" weaken them dramatically over time- rebounding can be a powerful ally in reversing this atrophy- rebounding is wonderful for restoring foot health and fitness.

For me, doing my virtual resistance exercises while also bouncing is combining the best of both worlds! You just bounce along, doing the high shoulder reach for reps, flexing your arms and shoulders as you continue gently bouncing... then hold and give an isometric hold! Repeat for maybe 7 reps, then go to the forward fly...

You go through the whole cycle of your body, methodically, while getting a rebounding workout in at the same time! In addition, your balance is dramatically improved from day #1, and even the flexes themselves are more intense because of the constant shift in your gravitational pull as your bounce!

I hope you are convinced that rebounding is something you should adopt?

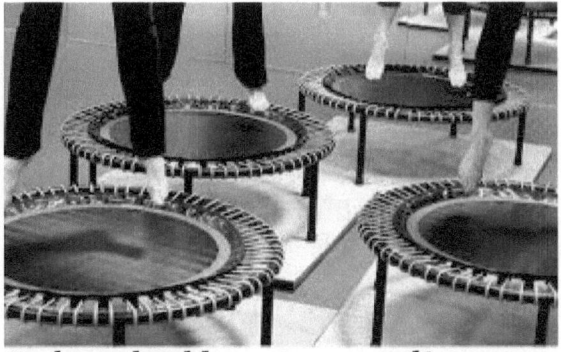

So, how should you get started?

You can go high end- the Bellicon, Reboundair, and Cellercizer- all are fantastic, Mercedes Benz versions of the rebounder!

But, you can do just fine, at least at first, with a cheap, simple rebounder for, oh, $36 dollars or so... way cheaper than good running shoes! (And it'll last a lot longer- and do WAY more good than those "cast-like" shoes!)

Just do it BAREFOOT for maximum benefit!

Go ahead- go on Amazon, or Target or Walmart- they all have rebounders! They're not great- but they will all WORK GREAT. Or, go high end- your choice.
If you've got the money, definitely- get a Bellicon, Reboundair, or Cellercizer- you do get what you pay for. But I want you to know that even a CHEAP rebounder will get you healthy, and start you on the road to detoxing your lymph system, and energizing your virtual resistance exercise in a Big Way!

#

TRAIN YOUR FEET, YOUR NECK, AND YOUR EYES

Most people do lip service to exercise, since everyone knows (at last!) that physical exercise is vital to health and wellness. Most older people, however, just walk at the mall, in highly cushioned shoes, or walk on a treadmill or around their neighborhoods- again, in highly cushioned walking shoes that are guaranteed to put your feet into a foam "cast", and thus make them ever weaker.

In terms of health and wellness, if your feet are in constant pain and discomfort, who cares what your 10K time is, or how much you can lift? Work out for a lifetime, I say, and that means first taking care of the basics!

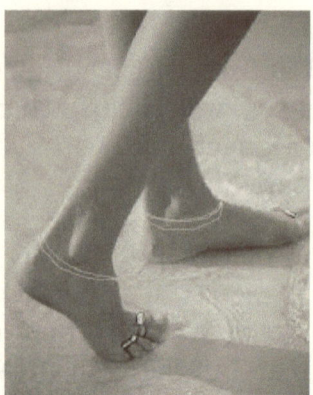

Every morning, during my Perfectly Paleo Exercise routine, I do several exercises especially for my feet! In addition, since I always work out barefoot in the living room, and wearing my Xero sandals when in the basement, my feet are constantly involved in whatever exercise I am doing, stabilizing with my toes, strengthening my arch, and twisting and bending as they are meant to do! And, I also massage my feet with my hands, routinely, as part of my workout. It doesn't take long, but the results are so worth it... even my hands and fingers are strengthened by that massage!

* * *

100

In warmer weather, I sprint once per week in the yard, barefooted. 5 or 6 hundred yard dashes or so, sometimes longer, for maybe 10-15 minutes. But build up to this! Start by just walking around your house either barefoot or in stockinged feet- never wear shoes in your house!

OK- that's your feet, becoming their paleo, healthy selves for a lifetime! Now, on to your neck...

The neck is the other part of the body that, when it hurts or is unnaturally weak, will really ruin your life! Think about the last time you had a sore or stiff neck- you couldn't do anything physical at all. So, during your daily morning workouts (I suggest working out daily, or almost daily for at least a short while) take some time to manually resist moving your head against your hands- push your forehead against your resisting palms, then backwards, and then from side to side. Push with perhaps a 70-80% perceived maximum resistance level, for a few seconds duration each way- that's it! It doesn't take long at all, and can really make a long term impact on your health- do you really want to be one of those elderly people that is permanently hunched over?

So, you've saved your feet, and you've saved your neck! Now, how important to you are your eyes??

It's not widely known, but the eyes are like the feet- use them naturally, as they are meant to be used, and they will become stonger! If you constantly wear eyeglasses or contact lenses, your eyes are essentially locked in casts- the will become weaker and weaker over time.

Don't wear your glasses indoors, unless you really, really need to. Hold books out to where you can barely read them, at the edge of your focus, and read them there. Don't make the print on your computer so BIG that it looks like the first

101

letters on an optometrist's eye chart- make your eyes work.

And above all, make a habit of looking off into the distance, and then back at something close up, and then back into the distance- exercise your eyes. Consider getting a weaker prescription, not a stronger one next eye Dr. appointment. Go to a behavioral optometrist, where they believe as I do- they will work with you to get gradually weaker prescriptions to strengthen your eyesight. A standard optometrist will try to sell you on a stronger prescription, with expensive lenses and frames each and every time you visit them.

It's a great business model for them, just like selling prescription drugs is great for the drug companies... but it will make your vision progressively worse. Just as the prescription drugs will mask the symptoms, while making your health progressively worse.

So treat the cause! Don't walk with cushioned shoes, which lead eventually to a cane, and then a walker. Go the other way- to LESS technology- walk barefoot! Exercise your feet.

Exercise your neck, and while you're at it, your spine and the rest of your body via Perfectly Paleo Exercise. Be physically healthy the rest of your life- try going glasses free as much as possible too!

We were created to be perfectly functioning humans. We evolved to match an environment that we have unwittingly turned toxic, through too much ease and comfort on the one hand, and too much stress and unnaturalness on the other- toxic city water loaded with chemicals, endless job responsibilities, outrageous taxes and overbearing government control.

We need to go back as much as possible! Our future is in our past.

Try to live in the real world, the paleo world. Anything else is madness.

#

IF YOU **DON'T** HAVE TIME FOR EXERCISE, YOU **WILL** HAVE TIME FOR DISEASE!

Heed this advice- you DO need to exercise! Not super hard, and to "failure" as so many recommend- definitely NOT.

But, your body was definitely built to MOVE, and if you don't move around, a LOT, you will definitely be making room for disease, and your life will be shorter, and FAR less pleasant than it could be otherwise.

Diet, of course, is important. Vitally important!! So, with that in mind, grasshopper: cut out the processed foods, the fast foods, the sugar, and above all the grains! The grains are the hardest for everyone, since they've been touted, pushed, lauded, and applauded for decades!

BUT THEY ARE POISON TO YOUR BODY AND MIND!!

That's it, that's the bottom line: if you didn't know before now that our own American government, medical clinics, and so-called "leaders" have been lying to you...

Well, now you do.

The "food pyramid", or now the "my plate" promoted by your tax supported government agencies-

Is guaranteed to make you sick, fat, diabetic, and prone to heart disease and cancer!

Multiple servings of grains and sugars per day will do that.

103

So, cut that out, and go back to the diet of your grandparents. Eat real food, meat and veggies, real fat (nothing of vegetable "fake" fats like margarine or soy oil- just real foods, like God made them!!

GMO grains are made to be avoided. Who wants to be part of a government experiment to see if maybe these will kill us, but we won't know for years??

But back to topic: EXERCISE. You need to do it. Your body's genetic expression expects it, and if it doesn't happen, your whole body will start to unravel- give up- it actually thinks it is already DEAD.

Our bodies NEED movement, and they need physical exercise, or stress!

Start out with pushups, and walking barefoot.
I
f you can do 20 pushups, start out with ten. If you can do 10, start out with 5. If you can't do any, do them supported on your knees "Girl pushups, if you will", and do one or two.

It doesn't matter where you start- the important thing is to progress, gradually. Your body will thrive on this! All it wants is a direction- either towards health, fitness, and wellness...
or towards less movement, less vitality, disease and death.

Your body, and Nature doesn't really care, either way-
It is YOUR CHOICE.

I have chosen movement, and health, fitness, and wellness! I start each morning, and I recommend you do as well, with virtual resistance exercises, followed by intensive stretching, and then PUSHUPS.

Just like (I hope!) you learned in grade school, as I did.

As I said: start out with about one HALF of the amount you can do. Do NOT go to failure, or anywhere near failure!

Then, after a brief rest, do another set of one half what you can really do! (I do mine in front of the TV, so this is really not onerous at all)- I limit my TV watching to when I am exercising, so I really look forward to it.

You will too, if you observe this caveat!

I don't care how advanced, or unadvanced you are, physique-wise... this system works amazingly well for anyone!

You do the exercise (please be sure to use perfect form), and NEVER go to failure, or even CLOSE to failure. Repeat.

Repeat again.

Keep repeating.

Watch the show. (I am currently watching *"Longmire"*, which I love!) Your taste may vary.

As you watch, feel your muscles, how they move- concentrate on the feeling of movement, like an animal would. And just keep repeating, over and over, pushups after pushups- trust me, it's kind of pleasant, gives you a feeling of accomplishment, and it flushes most of the major muscle groups of your body with life-giving blood!!
This is an incredibly health giving exercise routine, and over time will literally transform your physique, your health, and your life!

Ironically, since it really isn't all that hard, once you get in the morning habit, it's really....simple, easy, and actually enjoyable- something you'll actually look forward to!

And believe it, you will gradually get stronger and stronger, slowly, and injury free. You won't need to spend any extra money on arcane training programs, supplements, or anything at all!

To sum up, here is what you need to do for maximum health and wellness:

Eat real foods! (God and Nature made foods, that we evolved to eat and thrive on).

Avoid modern grains, sugars, and processed foods! (Anything labeled low fat is particularly BAD).

Exercise: Spend at least 20 minutes each morning, watching television and doing pushups, stretching, and otherwise "getting in touch with your physical being!"

Last, and probably MOST importantly-
WALK!

Slowly is fine, probably better than a herky-jerky fast motion. The best walking is done barefoot, or at least with minimal shoes like moccasins, or Xero shoes, that do not have raised heels, and allow your feet to move naturally. This is great for not only your foot health, but also your knee, hip and ultimately your spine health!
There is a lot about how many "steps" you need to take, I don't think this is valid: just make an effort to walk.

Park really far at the grocery, or the big box stores! It only takes seconds to walk past the crowded, packed in cars that all are obsessed with getting as close as possible to the entrance!

And take "forest bathing nature walks" as often as possible! Nothing is more restorative, both to body and mind, as walking, ideally barefoot, on a pristine path through a forest, or along a beachfront.

If you can do it daily, do it! Otherwise, just do it as often as you can.

Not only your physical health, but your mental health depends on it.

Paleolithic Philosophy!

SCRIPT OUT YOUR MORNINGS!

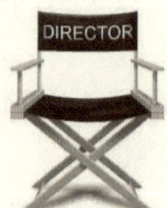

The thing about waking up, and starting your day to remember is that it is the most important part of your day, and so of your life! What you do to start your day actually determines your DAY- the outcome depends upon the beginning!

Especially with health and wellness, this is crucial. First, you need to start a good, productive, happy day with a really good night's sleep- and that is super important!!

Ok, I guess your perfect day starts with going to bed nice and early; enough to get a good 8 hours or so of quality, blacked-out room quality type of sleep...
But now, it's morning! Do NOT lay in bed thinking about all the things you should do, or not do- go to your scripted, pre-planned, programmed every day morning routine:

I have one, that works very well for fitness, health, productivity, and overall HAPPINESS! Want to hear it? OK:

I awake, just before my alarm clock. Always! I get up quite early, before work so I can do my script! After all, it IS the most important time of my day!

I start in by doing deep breathing, deep costal breathing-meaning that I breathe deep into my diaphragm, swelling my abdomen with life-giving oxygen,and then fill my chest as well to the max, and then slowly exhaling until my lungs are completely empty. Repeat.

Do this maybe 10 times or so, and you are completely awake, and energized! The benefits of this total costal breathing are wonderful, and not to be underestimated.

Then, I arise and go into the bathroom, where I do a series of limbering moves- not really "exercises", but just moves where I take my limbs and joints, slowly and easily, through a range of motion to get them activated.
Shoulders, neck, elbows, knees, hips, and ankles... Maybe 3 minutes or so.

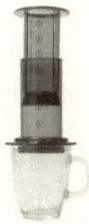

Aerobie Press

Then, I go downstairs, and heat up water for coffee in an electric carafe for coffee. I add coconut oil to three cups, about a teaspoon or so, and then, when the water is hot, I make the organic coffee with my wonderful Aerobie Press coffee maker! (This is the best way to make coffee- better than machines that cost thousands of dollars- trust me!) And, whilst the water is being heated, I take the canister from my trusty Vitamix Blender and load it up to make my own food supplements for the next few days!
I start out with about a cup of green tea, which I pretty much always have in my kitchen thermos, and a can of coconut milk...

* * *

And then, I begin adding in: kefir, spirulina, kelp, cinnamon, ginger, turmeric, spinach, the frozen california mix of veggies... heck, just check out my perfectly Paleo smoothie recipe at www.paleojay.com and you will be golden! With this elixir of the gods made in my Vitamix, I have achieved my nutritional script for the next few days, and cannot fail- I have reached nutrition NIRVANA!!

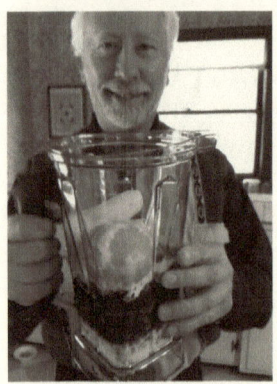

Next, I take my perfect cup of coffee into the living room, and turn on Netflix...

This is pretty much the ONLY time I watch TV- when I exercise!

I turn on my latest compelling movie or news program, and begin my virtual resistance exercise, which is flexing intensely while you move through a total motion. It achieves all that I used to get through weight training, but with no damage to joints and tendons, and much more naturally and pleasantly! It is the cornerstone of my fitness regimen, and I recommend it to everyone- weight training and Aerobics are the USDA Food Pyramid of exercise- those forms of exercise are highly recommended, almost universally so, yet their results lead inevitably to injury and debilitation!

* * *

Just as the food pyramid, or My Plate update of the stupid Food Pyramid leads to obesity and disease nutritionally!

Moral of the story? Anything recommended by Big Government, Big Food, or Big Anything is a LIE, meant to benefit THEM!!

I hate tattoos, but if you must get one, that would be worthwhile...

OK, back to the script: You have spent maybe 15 enjoyable minutes exhausting the muscles of each part of your body, methodically, in turn, while you were engaged watching a television program you really wanted to watch! Not a bad way to start your day, is it?

NOW, do the same thing, but do it on your rebounder! You know, the little mini trampoline you bought on Amazon? Just get a cheap one at first- they are fine; later you can upgrade to a Bellicon- but the cheap ones ($50 or so) work well enough.
You just slightly bounce (you're still watching TV remember) while you go through your same Virtual Resistance exercises that you learned at www.paleojay.com, or at www.transformetrics/exercises.com.

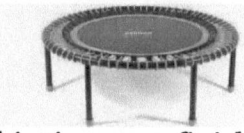

But this time, you finish each move at a different ending point:
half-way up, or all the way up, or at the beginning of the movement.

And, when you finish, you hold it isometrically, for several seconds.

This makes a huge difference in the results- that isometric hold!

I like to start with first cycle, hold in the beginning part of the motion (say the beginning of the curl), second part on the rebounder in the middle, and the third motion at the end of the movement! And, since you are bouncing throughout, you are simultaneously exercising and energizing every part, and every cell of your body.

Now, I don't do the same routine every day, and neither should you. But this is my base routine, my home place that I do pretty much on a daily basis.

And if you have a base routine, a script that you follow, and don't even have to think about, daily...

Well, welcome to health, wellness, and happiness!

It's all built in. After this, everything else is strictly downhill.

#

Is Paleo "Barbarian"?

Are we, as followers of the paleo diet, more like this dying Gaul below than the civilized Romans?

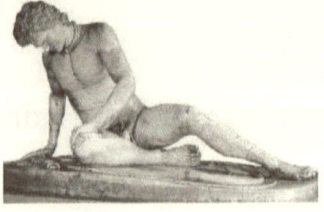

Let me throw some ideas your way:

From what I've been able to glean, the Gauls were primarily

meat and dairy eaters.

They also raised grain, and used a good bit of it to make beer- a beverage that the wine drinking Greeks and Romans found disgusting. They did also have bread, and porridge made from grains and lentils, but from all indications this was kind of "back burner" food- the preference of these tribal barbarians was for meat, cheese, and butter, of which they had quantities available; both from the widely available hunting, and the herds they kept.

They also had vegetable gardens, but of course the white potato was unknown. The northlands they dwelt in had not been overgrazed, which was the case around the Mediterranean, the erstwhile "Fertile Crescent", which had been overgrazed for centuries since the dawn of civilization there, and was beginning to gradually turn to desert.

The Romans were a largely predatory civilization, and had become rather puny physically over time compared to the barbarian Gauls... they were victorious over the Gauls and others not from physical superiority, but through a specialization of warfare technique that made each soldier function as a cog in a giant machine of disciplined warfare, rather than using individual initiative.

Here is a good description of the diet of the Romans around the time, 2nd Century BC, that our gladiator friend above lived (and died) in:

The lower class Romans (plebeians) might have a dinner of porridge made of vegetables, or, when they could afford it, fish, bread, olives, and wine, and meat on occasion.

Since many of the lower class were citizens, the ancient Romans had a program to help them, somewhat like a welfare program. The welfare program was called the annona.

There was also a separate WIC-type or school-lunch program (the alimenta), just for kids, which was instituted, or at least greatly developed in early 2c CE.

In the regular food welfare system, people were issued welfare stamps, which were little tokens, called tesserae. How these were issued (remember there was no open public postal system), and how Romans identified themselves to the authorities in the first place, we do not know. You showed up with your tokens (tesserae) and containers, at large government warehouses. You got wheat flour -- or bread already baked from government bakeries, and other foodstuffs. Meat was distributed on special occasions with special tokens."

This is interesting, not only in the rather Paleo type diet of the Gauls, and the modern, civilized, grain based diet of the Romans, but in the social governmental control being used by the Roman government in its "dole", or Welfare system. Perhaps it is an inevitable development of civilization to use low quality food as a means to control their populations?

Here is a quote from the seminal science fiction author Philip K. Dick:

"We live in a society in which spurious realities are manufactured by the media, by governments, by big corporations, by religious groups, political groups. I ask, in my writing, What is real? Because unceasingly we are bombarded with pseudo-realities manufactured by very sophisticated people using very sophisticated electronic mechanisms. I do not distrust their motives. I distrust their power. It is an astonishing power: that of creating whole universes, universes of the mind. I ought to know. I do the same thing."

To me, this sounds like a description of the current state of affairs between Big Government, Big Pharma, and the Big Processed Food manufacturers- manipulating us with sophisticated marketing, selling us fake, non- nutritional foods that

1. Keep us misinformed
2. Keep us sick
3. keep us addicted to the foods they sell that make us sick
4. Keep us reliant on expensive drugs that they sell

I've always revered and loved the glory that was Greece and Rome. But now, I'm starting to think rather often of a quote from the author Robert E. Howard, from his most popular hero Conan the Barbarian-

"Barbarism is the natural state of mankind. Civilization is unnatural. It is a whim of circumstance. And barbarism must always ultimately triumph."

What do you think? Am I a little paranoid here, or not?

\#

YOUR FAMILY IS YOUR MOST IMPORTANT TRIBE

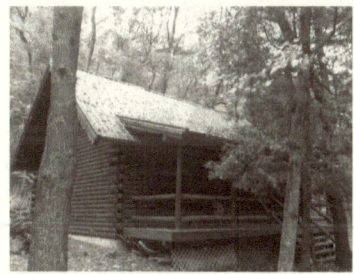

NEW CABIN ROOF!!

I just got back, this morning from a whirlwind connection with my familial tribe.
95 yr. old father, year born unknown mother, and assorted brothers, nieces and nephews...the connections are diverse, and definitely not of the daily variety, but they are all-family!

I had gone down to Illinois to help my brother clear out an overgrown woods at his new house and acreage with my new chainsaw. (My old one was just worn out, having done more in its 10 year life than ever should have been expected of it!) My new, 20" bar chain saw wasn't cheap, but I will say it was a Stihl...

Anyway, as we worked, clearing the logs and fallen trees from a creek in the back of his property that had been overgrown and neglected for about 30 years, we were doing what has been done by man since time immemorial- working together, as a tribe, accomplishing real physical work that really needed to get done. And as we worked, other relations all showed up, and then, it was time for a celebration of sorts- we drove over the river and through the woods, to grandpa and grandma's we'd go!

It was fun to connect with my little nieces and nephews, not to mention my little brothers, when we all got there. It's funny how many old memories are rekindled, how many shared laughs from the past are in our minds, as if experienced only yesterday!

One nephew wanted to see Grandma and Grandpa's old photo albums, and really laughed when he saw old photos of his dad as a kid, and of me when my hair wasn't white as the snows of Mt. Olympus!

* * *

PaleoJay's Smoothie Cafe!

Now, traveling can be exciting and diverting, but it can also make it hard to remain paleo, even if you have convinced SOME of your family to also "get on board". Food is the hardest part: the best solution is to, as I did, pack a generous lunchbox full of
Paleo Smoothie! A proper, paleo type of smoothie, as I outline in detail on www.paleojay.com, and in this very book!

I say a proper smoothie because, a real smoothie is made by you, at home in your Vitamix blender, not purchased at a Smoothie Bar, or bottled by a manufacturer!

The reason for this caveat? The smoothie you make yourself is the very healthiest, most nutrient dense nutrition possible for your body to consume. The other, "bought 'en" version are loaded with useless sugars, too much fruit, not enough fiber, and concentrate totally on taste, and hardly any at all on nutrient density!
Each morsel you consume should go to further your body's ability to repair, regenerate, and revitalize itself! Anything else just drags you down.

So, I packed canning jar after canning jar of Paleo Smoothie in my giant lunch box, along with a cold pack..

Next, put in ample amounts of snacks, like almonds mixed with dark chocolate chips, celery with almond butter on it, an apple, macadamia nuts, well- any nut but a peanut, which is a legume! If you have been paleo for any length of time, you know what to pack!

I always include a couple of tins of sardines. If you are really hungry, nothing is better for you than these little fish, since you are consuming the whole carcass- the bones, the organs (like the liver!)- this is really one of the most nutrient dense foods on the planet.

And so, you get the idea- it is way easier to prepare, and not be misled by temptations when you are perfectly full already. It also saves you a lot of money!

Another way to cope is by just intermittently fasting or IF. This is simply compressing you "eating window" into a smaller block of time, i.e. rather than 3-6 meals (and snacks!) per day, just eating two, or even one meal a day, and fasting or skipping one meal. Most Paleo Gurus recommend skipping breakfast, perhaps having some Paleo coffee, which is just fat mixed in your coffee, to give you a ketogenic head start to the day. I like coconut oil and heavy whipped cream, topped with cinnamon and cloves, but that's just me- you may prefer Dave Asprey's Bulletproof coffee, which is MCT oil and grass fed butter mixed in your coffee, or Mark Sisson's Primal Egg Coffee.

Which is, you guessed it, eggs in your coffee! I think a much better, but similar version is to heat up a mug of bone broth, and stir in a scrambled egg- instant super healthy egg drop soup!

Me, I guess I'm just not a true Paleo Guru- I like to skip supper instead, and so, after my morning Paleo Coffee of coconut milk and cream, which I like to sip as I work out ala Perfectly Paleo Exercise, and also as I drive to work after a big breakfast. I include my Paleo Smoothie in my breakfast, and also throughout my work day in my big lunch box, packed in wide mouth canning jars, and made fresh in the morning in my big Vitamix blender.

I also pack a big lunch, often a big salad, topped with meat or seafood, hard-boiled eggs, lots of greens, sometimes anchovies, avocado, and real olive oil based dressing- YUM!
* * *

PaleoJay's Smoothie Cafe!

Oh, as far as the coffee goes, I think coconut oil and cream are enough- I put a slab of butter right in the smoothie, along with a couple of raw pastured eggs! All bases covered; well, isn't that what a Paleo Smoothie is all about??

Supper time rolls around, but I am not hungry for supper, most nights! One less meal to plan, and clean up from, and steal time from your hobbies and projects and music and neighborhood tribal connections...

But, when I travel, sometimes I do it the Paleo Guru way- Coffee with fat in it in the morning, big lunch and/or smoothie later in the day, and dinner that evening- I mean, if I'm just traveling in the AM, why stop for a meal? Get there, then eat AND socialize!

Then you can be a really good tribal member! Hurrah Paleo Peep!

Also, you may be tempted to pack or buy enroute Paleo Products- bars, potions, all kinds of convenience products. Although OK occasionally, it is much better to just eat real food, all of the time!

My brother packed me, instead of sandwiches for the return journey, swiss cheese and salami rolls! They were so good when driving, and quite satisfying and nutritious...

And, the day I drove down, I had a smoothie in the morning in the car, and then a bowl of chili that evening- so, that day, I skipped lunch!

There are so many ways to tackle IF, you can mix and match them, but I stand with my favorite: Skip Supper!

* * *

119

The other problem when traveling and visiting is sleep! This one is huge, and the hardest one of all to cope with, I think. Strange beds, people interacting constantly...
And did you know that people with inadequate sleep, or those that work shift work jobs, increase their cancer risk by 5 times!?

The best rule is to just get to bed as early as you can! Then, you can get up before everyone else, ideally, and even go for a walk, meditate, or even do a little visualized resistance, or at least your daily warmup for your joints and muscles before you are distracted by the activities of the day.

So, go ahead and connect with your TRIBE! Eat well and ancestrally, teach them all by your example and level of fitness. Help out with projects! And then, head home knowing that your tribe is all around you, in spirit if not in fact, and that in every real respect they are really, truly a part of you.

Then, if you are like me, your ever-faithful PaleoJay, you will head home, but stop at your family cabin to... do more chain sawing! yikes!! A big storm had dropped a giant tree on our cabin, punching a hole in the roof, and necessitating a new, green metal roof replacement! Glad about that metal part...

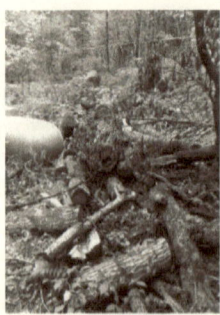

Lots and LOTS of logs and branches to cut and stack, and

drag and pile... Another long afternoon, this time by myself. But, in my mind, the whole tribe was there,enjoying the grounds as they will in the future, benefiting from my labors. That makes it all more than worthwhile!

#

BARBARIAN FITNESS AND NUTRITION

Another designation I have always had for Paleo Quick Start nutrition and exercise is "barbarian fitness".

I know that this just makes people think somewhat negatively about the concept: I mean, weren't barbarians just stupid, and not really "civilized"?

Well, that's right, in a way... they were open to the advantages of civilization, but were also well aware of the weaknesses of civilized living. Barbarians, in their best sense, have been paleolithic tribal people who also took advantage of the technologies developed by civilized folks when those technologies were to their advantage.

Think of barbarians as living on the "outskirts" of ancient civilizations; primarily Rome. Germanic tribes were predominant, but there were others; the Celts, the Thracians- many others.

I imagine that they respected the civilized achievements of those Romans, but were highly suspect of the other, what they would have seen as decadent aspects of that same civilization!

I think we, as Paleo folk, are kin to the barbarians:

Living on the outskirts of a civilization that we realize has become... decadent.

121

Poisoning the environment, lacking in morals, even eating foods that are sadly lacking in the nutrition needed by vital, active humans- barbarians are willing to AVAIL themselves of the benefits of civilization, but are also all too aware of the drawbacks of the lifestyle- the Neolithic grains, the relinquishing of basic human rights to an aristocracy and priestly class- the subservience of civilized stratified life!

 So, as "barbarian fitness" practitioners, we should imagine ourselves as living "on the edge" of a corrupt empire, taking advantage where we can from it's bounty, but also cutting ourselves off from the many corrupt shortcomings that have settled into it's workings...

Take the BEST of civilization, and PRESERVE the best of our hunter/gatherer forebears_

This is the role of the BARBARIAN!

To take the best of both worlds. A kind of hunter/gatherer-civilized person amalgam.

And, speaking of taking advantage of the best way of doing things, let's talk about sculpting your body- weights and machines are the best way, right?

Wrong! This is another case of civilized thinking getting it wrong- machines isolate individual muscle planes of motion, and build mostly just bulk. Free weights, while a better option, also primarily build muscle bulk, and they both ignore tendon and ligament strength.

What you need to develop is the all -important mind-to-muscle connection- that is what really lets you tense and develop the musculature with symmetry and proportion- this enables you to cultivate the look and athletic function of a classic greek athlete, not the unhealthy bulk of a 300 pound lineman, Olympic or power lifter...

 The very best, and most accessible option for maximum safety and optimum results for both men and women is visualized resistance!

You'll almost never hear this talked about, simply because, just like the Paleo/Ancestral/Primal/Barbarian diet- there is nothing to sell!

You just tense the muscles of your body, methodically, throughout their complete range of motion, kind of a "flexing meditation" that you perform through each plane of motion in turn, until your whole body has been stretched, renewed, and stimulated to grow and shape itself in the very best way for your own genotype!

Sounds too good to be true, I know, but it really is the best thing since sliced brea---, uh, no, I mean since grass finished beef liver on the grill with hollandaise sauce!

Just add in some bodyweight exercise to finish- pushups, chin ups, straight legged sit ups, hindu pushups and hindu squats, and finally some sprinting once a week or so...

 You will naturally develop your body to it's own God given potential, and most NATURAL, appealing, and functional state.

 So- eat like a barbarian, train like a barbarian, and you will look, feel and perform like a barbarian! And that is definitely a positive!

Movement is Life!

TIDY UP YOUR LIFE AND YOUR HEALTH

I recently read a book called "The Life-Changing Magic of Tidying Up- the Japanese art of decluttering and organizing" by Marie Kondo.

This was actually a revelation of a book to me- in this slim volume (only about 200 pages) is a well organized prescription of just how you can totally organize your living space and all of your possessions! It is a strange sort of book choice for me, since I didn't even think I needed to go through my clothing, my books, and actually everything I own...but my daughter, and a couple of friends highly recommended it, and so I did.

And I am so glad that I did!

I am not a really cluttered person, but like in everything, there is always room for improvement. I started with my outdoor shed, which is attached to my garage and just loaded with stuff- since it's winter here in Wisconsin, I waited for a warm-ish day, and then began- I took everything out, and then, after adding a home made workbench made from old bathroom cabinets and a heavy duty slab of pressboard for a top, put it all back...perfectly ordered and with everything available, and MINUS all of the other stuff that resided there.

I would take Marie's advice, and hold each item in my hands, and ask myself if I needed it, or truly wanted it, or ever thought I'd use it again. If it was perfectly good, but I

124

thought I'd never use it again, I thanked it in my mind for serving me, but now it was time to let it go. I got rid of so much junk, and in just a matter of several hours had a delightful workspace, even with the storage of many summer items like tillers, mowers, rakes, shovels, hoes, etc. etc.- all neatly organized and easily accessible.

I had "turned Japanese" like the old Cheap Trick song from the 1970's, and was now enamored of tidying!

I moved on to my closet, and learned to make decisions about every item of clothing I owned, and threw out very, very many things that were basically just encumbering me with useless, cluttered storage. I learned to fold my t-shirts, shirts, handkerchiefs, socks, and everything else properly, and not ALL of my clothing items are available at a glance- nothing is stacked beneath something else, and every item is something I would really be sad at not having, and most importantly something that I can use and choose at a moment's notice. No searching or forgetting that something even exists anymore! It makes living on a daily basis simple and pleasurable.

And what does this have to do with out HEALTH? Actually, it is so similar in function that I couldn't stop relating the two even as I read the book. It is vitally important to our diet to clean out and dispose of every item in our cupboards or refrigerator that does not serve our health well!

Start with your cupboards- empty out your flour bin, your sugar bin- throw that crap OUT! I have potato starch (to feed my gut microbes in my Paleo smoothies) in the flour bin, and I keep green and white tea bags in my sugar bin. Go through your refrigerator- throw out anything that does not serve your HEALTH and well being- skimmed milk, anything low fat, industrial seed oils like margarine, corn, soy, canola, peanut oils- throw them away! Salad dressings made of these oils- do NOT hang onto them in the name of frugality- these things are you health's mortal enemies! Throw out anything made by man, and keep what is made by God.

Make sure you have PLENTY of good, Paleo types of real foods to eat, all neatly stored and easily accessible. To quote Marie Kondo in one of her best sayings: "The best way to find out what we really need is to get rid of what we don't" . This holds true for both possessions, and for foodstuffs!

And don't stop there- "tidy up" your exercise gear as well! If you have free weights and barbells- give, sell, or throw them away! You can keep a couple of light dumb bells, and should make or buy a good kettle bell- but other than these weights are a mistake! Heavy barbells and dumb bells can only compress your spine, gradually destroy your joints, and set you up for inevitable injury- heavy resistance is contraindicated for health.

In addition, weights are totally unnecessary for building your best strength and physique for your body type. Go with Virtual resistance exercise, self resisted (one limb resisting against the other as in curls being resisted with the other arm), and body weight exercise like pushups, pull ups, hindu and pistol squats. I still have all of my weights from years ago, and realize I have not touched them for over 8 years- in which time I have vastly improved my physique and strength levels from where I was at when I was 57, and at the same time totally healed my weight lifter's chronic knee, back, elbow, and shoulder problems!

Perfectly Paleo Exercise indeed! Just as we are not meant by God and nature to live our lives inflamed, fat, and subject to the myriad of modern, largely autoimmune- based diseases like diabetes, heart disease, obesity, and cancer, we are also not meant to live with painful or ruined joints, chronic pain, and physiques that are bloated travesties, with bulging abdomens and fat butts (from heavy squats), and woman like "man-boobs" from heavy benches, and the many back, knee, and shoulder problems that are inevitable with such heavy training.

So, you don't need a weight bench, squat stands, all the myriad of resistance machines and apparatus out there- get rid of them!

But, take this opportunity of newly available space and reduced clutter to get those few things that are really helpful and desirable to have in your lifelong quest for fitness- get your self a set of gymnastic rings to hang in your garage or basement, or even in your living room or to hang from a tree or playground structure. With just these alone, you can build quite a physique and high level of strength, easily and safely!

For my morning virtual resistance exercise, I had been using a towel on the living room carpet for years- I got myself a yoga mat, and it is a vast improvement for about $20! I don't need to use a pillow case to cushion my forehead on bridging anymore- also, it's great for the yoga-like stretches I include in my morning exercise ritual.

Definitely, you will want a rebounder! You don't hear much about these in the "serious" fitness community- but there is no safer, more accessible, and effective way to address your overall cardiovascular health than by putting one of these in front of your television! And vital for activating your lymph system for toxin and waste removal.

And the last thing I would add in the "Tidying Up" of your exercise equipment would be Perfect Pushup handles! Just the safest, most ergonomically correct and friendly way to do

127

your pushups, without putting strain on the joints of the wrist, elbows, and shoulders.

So there you go- declutter and tidy up! Not only in your house, and garage, but in your HEALTH!

WALK LIKE A MAN! (OR WOMAN)!

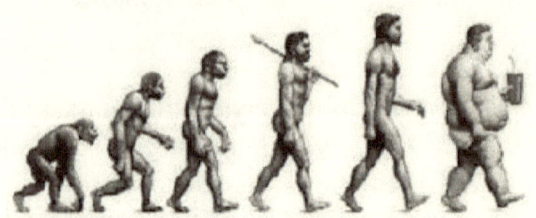

The guy on the right always parks right by the entrance...

I don't mean to be facetious, but here in Paleo Land, where all men are Conan, and all the women are Amazons, and of course all the children are not only above average but also birthed vaginally and loaded with good bacteria...

Walking is paramount!

Let's say all of your health markers are PERFECT! If you don't WALK, it is all for naught... your body will gradually shut down, thinking you must be dead...

This is literally true- if your human body, the ultimate achievement of our entire evolution perceives that you are a blob; that you are just sitting motionless in a cubicle or at a desk (or in front of your TV or Xbox) with only your fingers and eyeballs moving-

Your body knows you are DEAD- even if YOU DON'T!!

128

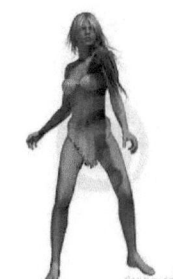

A Woman who WALKS!

Movement is literally LIFE, in evolutionary terms. Anything that is alive MOVES. Stop moving, and your very SELF gives up on you-

"Well" says your inner self, " I guess we're dead, or at least very near it. We must be locked in a cave, with tons of really bad food, but we must be dying slowly... I might as well shut down, and let the next generation take over, since I am obviously kaput, done, killed and ended!"

It doesn't matter if you are really enjoying yourself, eating pizza and watching TV at nights, and making big bucks driving around and in front of your computer selling gadgets and gizmos and then maybe working out on a treadmill for a 1/2 hour or so each day, followed by weights...

This is no life, and your body knows it- it knows you are DYING!

I watch animals, each and every day- birds, dogs, cats- and the one constant is constant movement! Not "training to failure" like weight training or Crossfit- not endless, chronic

129

cardio as Mark Sisson calls it, going into the "Aerobic Zone" and keeping it there as long as possible to "burn calories"...

Just simple walking, pure and simple. The most evolutionarily appropriate movement pattern for humans! Think about it: as infants, our primary goal is just to WALK!

We crawl, but as soon as we are able we get up, with assistance from walls and parents, but we get up AND WALK!

Walking barefoot is ideal, otherwise use minimal footwear like Xero shoes (which are really just a thin piece of rubber held beneath the feet, or moccasins; remember- shoes are casts for the feet. And anything put in a cast gets weaker and weaker...

This is our PRIME DIRECTIVE- WALK! All else is just frosting on the cake.

The true beauty of this is it's simplicity- walking is really the be-all and end-all of exercise! I started out many years ago with just WALKING. Then, when I got to age 20 I started lifting weights.

In my 40's, I gave up weights since I found them injurious, and went to Perfectly Paleo Exercise, which I deem to be Virtual Resistance (self resistance within the muscles) and bodyweight exercises.

Having regained the integrity of my joints by abandoning heavy weights, I now continue the Virtual Resistance exercises and pushups, pull ups, barefoot sprinting, and straight legged sit ups along with stretching on a daily basis- and I FEEL GREAT!!

* * *

130

PaleoJay's Smoothie Cafe!

I am now 63 years of age, and I plan to continue my daily regimen for my entire life. But you know what?

The mainstay of my fitness protocol is really just WALKING.

I walk around the yard (I have several acres) each day, barefoot; at least in the summer. I always park (to the chagrin of whoever is with me) at the VERY BACK of any parking lot when I go shopping!

My father, Phil Bowers, has always done this himself- ever since I can recall, he parked at the back of any lot, and we all walked to the store!

Other than this, and the fact that his favorite activities throughout his life were cutting, stacking and storing wood, gardening, and making music- the ultimate constant was constant MOVEMENT and walking!

I am going in July to visit my dad, to celebrate his 95th birthday. Luckily, he still lives in my childhood home, with my Mom, Carolyn, and they'll both walk out to greet me!

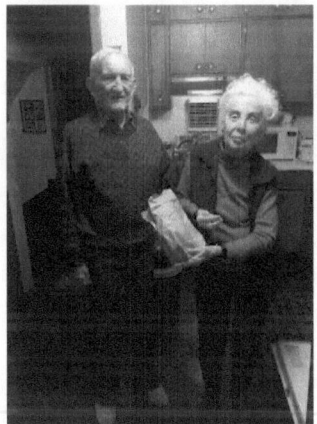

Phil and Carolyn Bowers at home!   * * *

131

HEAVY HANDS- THE BEST PALEO EXERCISE OF ALL

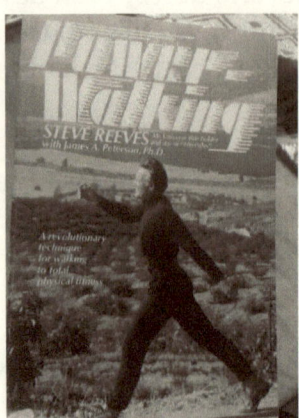

I was a heavy hands guy from the beginning, in 1982 I got Leonard Schwartz's book "Heavy hands", and it made real sense to me! I wanted to be aerobically fit, and I also wanted to be strong- before this I had jogged down our country roads for a few miles most days, and then lifted weights most other days...

It did work, quite well in most ways, but (this is my pre-paleo days!), my diet was sub-standard, and I started getting lots of aches and pains. My shoulders started aching from heavy bench presses (and other heavy lifts), and my knees and feet started hurting chronically as well from the running- remember, back then the running was "long and slow"- a perfect recipe for joint degeneration!

I also have a book by Steve Reeves, the classic era symmetrical bodybuilder, who came out with "Powerwalking" at about the same time! Steve had come up with a similar program, using small hand weights to up the

132

ante and exertion from walking, and they were both right on target.

Steve's book emphasized fast walking, while swinging hand weights as you go. Heavy Hands was more in depth, emphasizing the curling, and lifting of the weights more as you went, resulting in a real "Pan-Aerobic" exercise, as it was termed then.

Both are great concepts, but the Heavy Hands version wins out- you can mimic cross country skiing, arm and leg together walking exertion, and endless variations of multi-limbed exercise! I've always done it, periodically, since it is such a satisfying and result producing way of exercise, but now I am back in a big way!

I love to do my virtual resistance exercises, where the muscle provides its own resistance- (much better than weights, which injure your joints long term)! I do that each and every morning, along with stretching and calisthenics and then rebounding, right in front of my television... very relaxing and energizing!

My weights I have relegated to weighing down my tractor for increased traction, since I believe they create more harm than good in the long run.

Besides, bodyweight training yields actually better results!

But, each afternoon, I look forward to getting out my old heavy hands weights and handles, and walk down my forest paths pumping the weights in curls, and mimicking cross country motions, punching, pressing, and other motions that add to my walking exertion and spread it over my whole musculature.

It is like running with my whole body!

I love to sprint barefoot, and do in the warmer months every week, usually on Sundays. (It brings me back to my childhood, and burns fat faster than anything else, while strengthening my feet, and grounding me to mother earth at the same time).

But when I pick up my little dumb bells (8 lbs is about perfect for me) and walk down my forest trail, curling my arms alternately with each step, I realize that this is total body barefoot sprinting. Every part of my body is working at a high level of effort, but ironically- the perceived exertion level, i.e. the level of discomfort is markedly reduced!!

It is really hard exertion, but because it is spread across all the limbs (not just the legs) it seems much easier.

So, I can do it daily. I can do it barefoot. (Although, since it is getting colder here in Wisconsin I have started to wear my moccasins, which are really just like barefoot shoes, just not so obnoxious as those Vibrams with the toes...)

AND it exercises my entire body, as I move about and enjoy Nature and enjoy the sunshine, fresh air, pollen and other aspects of "Forest Bathing"!

And so, my final point is this:

If you had to choose ONE single exercise to stay healthy and fit:
I would go along with Steve Reeves, and Leonard Schwartz. Mr. Universe, and the psychiatrist.

Get some small dumb bells, pump them as you walk, and reap the benefits of Pan-Aerobics!

134

Jog with your whole body.

#

GREEN EXERCISE

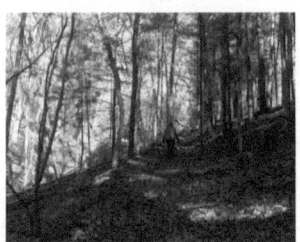

This is another name for something that I've been recommending for a long time now- I called it Forest bathing; where a person would walk about in nature, in a forest as I do almost daily, or in any natural landscape, be it a beachfront, along the river, or just in a park. It turns out that the University of Essex, in England, has been extensively studying the benefits of exercise in Nature for over 12 years!

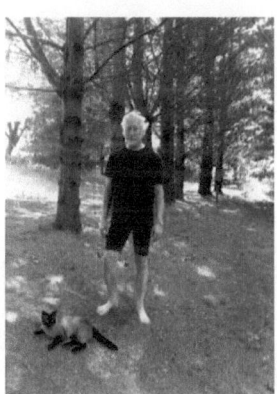

They have lots of studies that they have done on the benefits of exercising in nature as opposed to in a gym setting, and the benefits are manyfold. Primarily, mental benefits come from getting out in nature- just think about it, just as our paleolithic ancestors eating an ancestral, paleo type of diet, and we have evolved to do so as well- just as they slept long

135

hours each and every night- so too did they spent ALL of their waking hours out in nature!

It is something we have hard-wired into us. We are creatures of nature,and are meant to be IN nature on a daily basis. The best way to experience nature is by exercising outside, not just sitting in a chair, say, on a beach or in a lawn.
I like to take a hike through my woods on pretty much a daily basis. Barefoot is best, or now, when it is getting colder here in Wisconsin, I wear my Xero sandals, which are just a slim piece of rubber between my bare feet and the ground... later, when it's even colder, I will wear my moccasins, which are just leather between my feet and the ground, allowing my toes, and every tiny muscle in my foot to balance and strengthen as I go.

I think, beyond mental benefits such as alleviating stress and preventing depression and worry, such exercise has definite physical positives as well.

The hyper-oxygenated air in a forest or any plant covered terrain is wonderfully beneficial, as is the very sounds of nature: the rustling branches, the calls of birds and small animals, and the feel and crunch of pine needles and dry leaves underfoot. Even the pollen from the trees is something that is good for us, since we have co-evolved with it since before time began!

In addition, by being outside, we use our eyes as our ancestors did, as they are meant to be used. We look off towards the horizon, actively as we move, not at a screen right in front of our face, and we are engaged in, and actually a PART of nature! This is something we need reinforced, in this day of artificial,

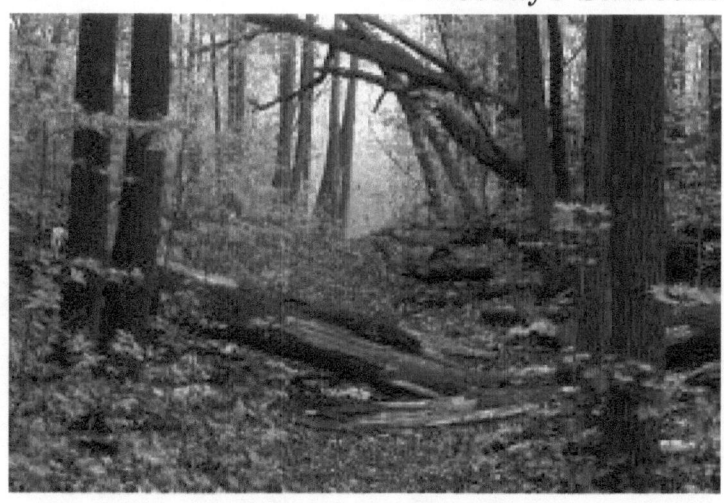

I sometimes, about once per week, sprint barefoot around my property, in short interval bursts. This is great, and something I look forward to, usually on Sundays.

But for a daily Green exercise regimen? Take a pair of small dumb bells, lately I've been using a pair of 8 pounders, one in each hand. Then PUMP them as you walk! This makes a leisurely walk, with plenty of time to observe nature as you go, into a demanding, total body workout.

Pump with high curls each step, or do side extensions for the deltoids as you go. Stop periodically, and do a set of pushups on the dumb bells- it keeps your hands clean, and you can go lower on each rep!

You can even stand perfectly still, and do curls, or presses for awhile, and then resume walking- a great variation is to mimic the moves of cross country skiing with the bells making the arms work as hard as the legs. Experiment! Have fun with this! It is demanding enough that it could be a stand alone exercise and mental health regimen.

PaleoJay's Smoothie Cafe!

Oh, it has a name, this dumb bell protocol- Heavyhands. It was very popular in the 1980's, and somehow has fallen out of the mainstream. I guess it is just so cheap and easy, so doable by anyone, that no one figured out how to make money off of it! (No expensive equipment, no pricey shoes or gym memberships)...

Oh- it also doesn't take long at all! 15 minutes is plenty; trust me, it's very taxing, but since all the "work" is spread around all of your limbs (PanAerobics), it seems easier.

So go ahead. Go green! Even if you're NOT a Packer's fan!

Flexibility is Key!

REBUILD YOUR EXERCISE DAMAGED BODY

I have said it before, and I will say it again: heavy weight training, endless cardio/aerobics sessions, and even the classic couch potato strategy all can, and usually do, result in the same result- an injured, weak, either just fat or "skinny-fat" body! They all come to the same, unintended destination- a physique that no one would want, with lots of damage, pain, too much fat tissue, and a predisposition to not ever do anything to aggravate the pain- which means no exercise at all- ever!

Obviously, this is a horrible conclusion. We all should resolve to be the adult that our 9 year old selves would have wanted!

We should all be fit and healthy, active and vital for our whole lives.
We should all remain as vital humans, who are proud of our bodies, proud of our physiques, and pleased with what we can do physically and mentally.
Pain free. Sleep well, and have no back, neck, hip, knee, or shoulder pain.
Strong, with a good endurance, and good flexibility.
Free of excessive body fat!
No chronic disease!!!

In the modern age, these seem to be increasingly elusive, if not impossible goals, at least in the public mind.

Everyone says things like "I'm too old now, I can't change."
And "I have to die of something!"

Here is the thing:

If you exercise with heavy weights, you will become injured.

No exceptions! I know, I've been there. Perfect form won't
save you. Low reps won't save you! Heavy weights, on a
regular basis, just aren't natural, they aren't "paleo", and
they aren't healthy!

Likewise, the endurance sports, like running, triathlon,
swimming and bicycling for distance and speed- will destroy
your musculature, your joints, and your health, setting you
up for cancer, fat storage once you stop (due to injury), and
endless pain in later life!

"Oh my GOSH!" you must be saying. "Why, maybe I should
just watch TV and play video games, be a couch potato and
save my body!!"

Sorry. That is the worst option of all! You will definitely get
back pain, and early on, and you are set on a collision course
with:
Diabesity, Mental fog, and an early demise!

SO WHAT SHOULD YOU DO??

Perfectly Paleo Exercise! It's really kind of a no-brainer, but
no one wants to consider it. You know- how pedestrian!
Bodyweight exercises? Pushups, sit ups, pull ups?
Simple stretches, self massage and back bridges??
Isometrics??? Self resistance???

And VIRTUAL RESISTANCE EXERCISE, where the muscles

generate the resistance internally, creating the same stress as heavy resistance but without the trauma?

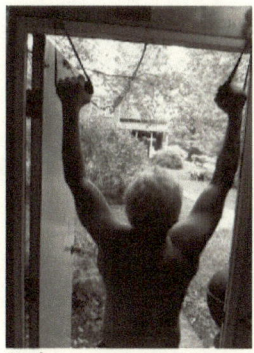

It just seems too good to be true. Especially since it has been common knowledge for thousands of years, throughout virtually every culture.

It's just not new and different!

Like Cross fit.

I'm kind of sad to bring this up, since the ideal of Cross fit seems so pristine...

But it's not, not at all. Cross Fit is a business, first and foremost. It had a great premise in the beginning: combine the various realms of fitness into a whole! Add in strength training, combine it with community and the spirit of competition and competitiveness, add in endurance and variety!

Wow- sounds great!

But then, they come up with Cross Fit "games". More competition! People pushing themselves... way too hard! Add in the pressure from that competition, multiply it to

"Win at all costs!", and we wind up with:

MASSIVE INJURIES.

OK- here is my bottom line:

Do not see fitness as a competition! It's not a race, it's not a contest, it's not the "Hunger Games"!
Just like proper diet, in other words a diet free of processed foods, grain fed

industrial meats, and fast foods and excessive carbs-

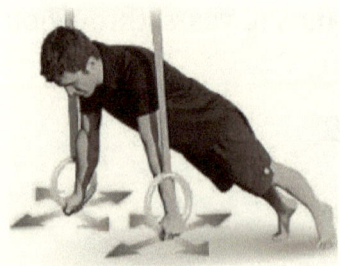

FITNESS AND HEALTH IS A WAY OF LIFE- NOT A COMPETITION!!

And this concept can be taken throughout your life. You can rebuild your damaged body- just do Perfectly Paleo Exercise!

Ditch the weights- throw away your running shoes- just do simple body weight exercise- in particular Virtual Resistance Exercise- this is the most rejuvenative of all!

Stretch and massage yourself as well. Just as proper diet is really simple, once you understand the basic principles, so is exercise!

Bottom line: Eliminate Wheat! And GET DOWN AND GIVE ME 20!!

(Or whatever- competition and pressure are irrelevant)

Just GIVE ME WHAT YOU HAVE GOT, AND STOP! THERE WILL BE MORE, TOMORROW!

Gradual, persistent, continual progression is the key. Kill yourself today, look good tomorrow, briefly, is irrelevant. And, winning an exercise competition is... counterproductive, and irrelevant!

#

THE VERY BEST EXERCISE EQUIPMENT, AND THE ONLY SAFE WAY TO DEADLIFT OR SQUAT HEAVY

I know, I generally say you don't need equipment to work out- after all, if you are doing virtual resistance training (flexing as you move through a muscles range of motion) and then holding isometrically... your own body is the resistance. And this is the most efficient and safe of all forms of exercise! It should be your warmup, and the core of your fitness regimen for the rest of your life. Nothing else even comes close in terms of totally working your entire physique! But it is also great to include other tools in your bodyweight arsenal. The first one I would recommend to you is the rebounder, or mini-trampoline.

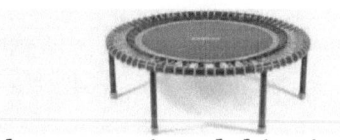

I have mentioned this piece of equipment before, and it is a wonderful addition to virtual resistance training- I often do

143

my virtual moving "poses" on the rebounder, usually in front of the TV...This kind of "doubles your pleasure, doubles your fun" in a good kind of way- you are working aerobically and your musculature at the same time. A really time efficient way to work out!

I am also a great fan of the pushup! And while the "hands flat on the floor" version is good, using a perfect pushup type of revolving handle is even better- not only does it raise your hands up off the floor, giving you a greater range of motion and more muscle engagement, it also protects your wrists and shoulders from damage by rotating along with the motion.

This protects your joints even as it makes the exercise more productive.

P bars, or parallette bars are another great option for pushups, giving you a VERY low extension point!

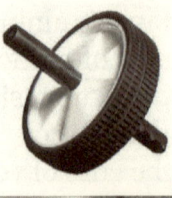

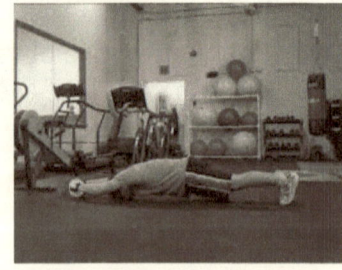

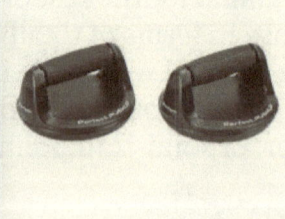

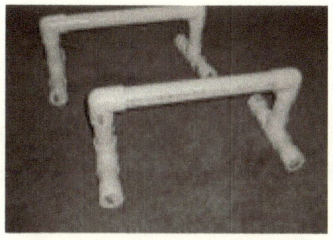

In a pinch, the perfect pushup device mentioned before can also be used for L sits! Just make sure you get the heavy duty version of the perfect pushup, as the other lesser version will wear out quickly supporting your body weight in the L sit, and doing pushups with your feet raised off the floor and resting on the back of a couch or chair while you do your leg raised of "Atlas 3" pushups.

An ab roller is wonderful, and actually another kind of pushup! Wonderful ab exercise, and it also simultaneously works the arms, chest, back and shoulders- also, it's a great party trick, as most men cannot do even one without gradually working up to it.

To begin, get an ab roller (they are quite cheap!) and do them from your knees. Next, you can do them from the top as a negative, going as slowly as you can downwards, and just stop at the bottom. Eventually you will get one full, top to bottom and back up again rep, and then you will add another, and another until you get to a set of 6 or 7. That's all you really need in terms of reps- then, just do multiple sets for a very high level of fitness! I like to "superset" ab roll outs with my sets of pushups.

Of course, a pull up/chin up bar is a necessity, but a tree branch of piece of pipe will do in a pinch.

I use my old power rack in the basement for this, back from my old weight lifting days of long ago, and a power rack or "cage" is a very versatile piece of equipment indeed- it is much more productive without weights, as it is ideal for isometric work, utilizing its pins to press against with empty bars or wooden dowels.

It is also great to use the power rack for squat variations- you can use the side supports to hold on to as you do a one legged or "pistol" squat. It helps to lean back as you do this, because that really takes the strain off of the knee joint and puts it right over the quadricep muscle where you want it. You can duplicate this upstairs, too, by doing these pistols in a door frame!

Another wonderful training adjunct is a set of gymnastic rings!

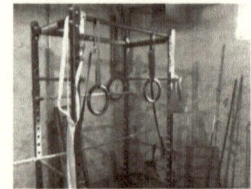

Now they are mounted on the ceiling joists!

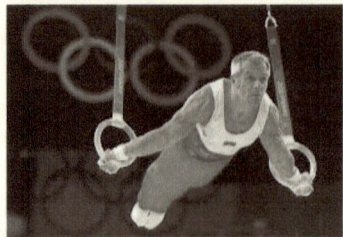

very advanced!

Mount these in your basement as I have, and you will find

146

them to be among the most satisfying, versatile and productive pieces of equipment you could possibly own.

They are wonderful to do pushups on! You can do Atlas 1,2,and 3 pushups quickly and conveniently, just by moving a little forwards or backwards to adjust the grips to be parallel to the floor (Atlas 1), angles halfway up (Atlas 2), or angled up high (Atlas 3).

They are also great for pull ups, L sits, and dips; also rows, and as assists for pistols!
Really- find a place for rings in your house, garage, basement or yard! They are just fantastic to train on.

I am saving the most crucial for last- an Exergenie is the ONLY way I recommend to do a deadlift, or a heavy squat!

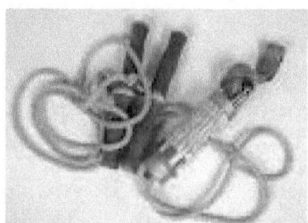

Exergenie

I know, this is controversial within Paleo Land, but it is also undeniable when you really look into it- just as gluten, and the other anti-nutrients in wheat and other grains are undeniably very harmful to human beings in their nutrition- so is lifting a heavy bar from the ground and standing up in a dead lift harmful to your back and other joints.

Also, putting a heavy barbell across your shoulders, and squatting, will compress your spine, inevitably damage your

147

knees, and set you up for serious, long-term injury.

And, it just gives you a fat butt, bulging abdomen, and blocky thighs- avoid these exercises!

High rep hindu squats, the aforementioned pistols, and the exergenie can give you anything these exercises can, BETTER!

I have an old exergenie that I bought off of Ebay- it has wooden handles, but they sell new ones too, and you can use it to do maximum effort deadlifts, squats, military presses, curls, and many other exercises. You feed the rope (that supplies the resistance) out with your fingers, and you can make the resistance as hard as you want throughout the whole range of motion. You can make it so hard that 3 reps is all you need for the squat and deadlift.

The best thing about the Exergenie is what you can do for your shoulders!

You can mount it in a door frame, closing the door on it 1/2 way up or so, and really lean into it, stretching out your shoulder girdle in every way possible. Then, you can pull back using just enough resistance to really work the entire shoulder region in every way- this is the very best way that I have found to really work the shoulders and protect the joint by strengthening both the muscles, tendons and ligaments gradually, from the inside out!

Along with a proper diet, and adequate sleep, these small pieces of training equipment can do far more for your health, strength, and physique than any gym membership you can name. And, you will have them forever, right in your living room or basement or garage, and can make maximum use of them for a lifetime!

#

GET **DOWN** WITH YOUR BAD SELF

One of the simplest, most important, and yet most ignored ways to improve your health, posture, flexibility is simply to spend more time on the floor!

Think about it: the simple chair or couch is the most unnatural, non-paleo way to support your body. It is taking a structure, and using it to support all of your limbs and musculature, encouraging a slouch and long term weakening of all the small supporting muscles throughout the body and spine. In particular, the muscles of the back and the butt are degraded the most over time- just look at most of our elderly population. They walk hunched over, with a permanent slouch, and their flaccid butts cannot even lift their feet very well off the floor.

This doesn't have to happen! Simply resolve to spend an hour per day or so on the floor. When I work out, about 1/3 of my exercise is spent on my mat on the floor, stretching, bridging, massaging my feet, doing straight legged sit ups, push ups, etc.
It is a mistake to always work out only in a standing position!

But, the bulk of your "floor time" can simply be hanging out, watching TV or reading, talking on the phone or to another person who is also on the floor! It's actually very "grounding" to be on the floor, and I don't mean that only in the literal sense. Being on the ground brings us back to when we were babies, before we even could get our selves off of the ground, or even roll over onto out backs!

But now, we need to maintain what we used to do effortlessly- do the Asian squat, as all toddlers do, to "sit" without a chair. This is actually the very best "exercise" you can do on a daily basis- just squat down and "rest" in a full, flat footed squat on the floor- and it isn't even really an exercise at all! This is the very best stretch for your back and legs of any you can possibly do- do it daily.

But actually, any way you sit or crouch or relax on the floor is good, much better for you than just sitting on the chair or couch. The transitions you make, moving from one floor position to another, and then when you stand, getting up smoothly from the floor under your own power- these are wonderful for your overall bodily health, utterly natural and necessary, and are so often lost to people by middle age!

Walking is important, but even more important is simply sitting on the floor, and being able to get up to a standing position easily and gracefully. To get up from a chair is like doing a squat down about a third of the way up- to get up from the floor is actually a rather complex, hinged motion involving the hand, arm, legs, hips, and back in a well coordinated and complex series of movements. It is very important that we maintain our ability to do this throughout life!

Asians have a largely floor based culture, and they are the better for it! When I was in Korea, I saw elderly folks get up from the floor after eating (this is how they traditionally dine) and they arose easily and smoothly. Even young Westerners often need to be helped up!

The chair is a cast! Think of it like that. The more you use a cast, the weaker you become. Eyeglasses are casts, shoes are casts- weaker prescriptions make your eyes gradually stronger, walking barefoot strengthens your feet and ankles. So strive to minimize using crutches of comfort to excess! Start by sitting on the floor- get DOWN with your bad self!

150

Medicine and Doctors!

YOUR DOCTOR CAN **NOT** SAVE YOU FROM A BAD LIFESTYLE AND DIET!

One of the biggest scams there is in this world is that conventional medicine, which is the kind of treatment you can get from an American clinic or hospital can make you WELL!

Nothing is further from the truth...a medical doctor of today just means that that person is a member of the biggest, most powerful labor union in history- the American Medical Association. This is a labor union par excellence- it guarantees incredibly high wages for the practitioners in "the Brotherhood" as Malcolm Kendrick calls it, as long as those doctors tow the line, don't rock the boat, and follow "approved" treatments ONLY- things like chemotherapy, radiation, and surgery only for cancer treatment- nothing else can even be considered, or the doctor doing so can be thrown out of the union- in other words -lose their high priced and time consuming right to practice medicine!

Your doctor is actually forbidden to recommend common sense lifestyle and diet changes to actually cure your condition, and is instead forced to recommend expensive pharmaceutical drugs (all of which have side effects, often worse than the disease!), and surgeries only. None of these options do any thing at all to address your disease or condition- they only mask the symptoms so you might feel a little better.

151

You will go home with your expensive prescriptions for drugs that make BILLIONS of dollars for the pharmaceutical companies annually, and billions of dollars for the medical clinic that prescribed them- all without curing your condition in the slightest.

You see, the pharmaceutical companies fund most of the research, and bankroll the medical colleges where the future M.D's train. They have a mutually beneficial relationship- the doctors recommend their products; in fact insist the patient use these products, and then everyone makes lots and lots of money... except YOU.

You are left sick, with endless pills and/or painful and damaging surgeries to endure, and are now a drug addict!

Even though your drugs are LEGAL, they are still usually endlessly necessary and actually addicting once you start, and hugely expensive- and, even though your medical insurance (if you have it) will mask the true costs since you only need a co-pay, rest assured that the ultimate cost is there, it is huge, and you are paying it through your other many taxes that are set to continue rising forever!

And let's talk side effects: All drugs have side effects!

This is often glossed over, but if you ever pay attention to the MANY drug commercials on the television all day long, listen to the potential side effects of the most popular ones, the ones they recite rapidly while showing attractive, loving couples dancing, walking on pristine beaches, and playing with laughing children and romping dogs: Here are the side effects of the Statin drugs, which are among the MOST prescribed drugs on earth!

* * *

152

Impaired liver function, muscle wasting and pain, possible heart attack risk, increased side effects with any other drug you might be taking, depression and irritability, headaches, joint pain, and abdominal pain, tingling, numbness and burning, sleep problems, sexual function problems, dizziness and a sense of detachment. Additionally, people have mentioned experiencing swelling, shortness of breath, vision changes, changes in temperature regulation, weight change, hunger, breast enlargement, blood sugar changes, dry skin, rashes, blood pressure changes, nausea, upset stomach, bleeding, and ringing in ears or other noises.

In addition, Statin drugs, which include Crestor, lipitor, and several other brand names tend to deplete CO q10, which is a vital substance manufactured by your body to produce cell growth and maintenance in every cell in your body- as you grow older, the supply lessens, and it can cause your heart to malfunction, and cause brain and cognition problems as well!

And all of those are from just one drug- most people, as they age and visit the doctor more frequently, are put on multiple drugs, which often have effects upon each other, independent of the drugs themselves. (Kind of like mixing heroin with cocaine and tequila, I'd imagine...)

I could go on and on about about the many, many drugs that literally are "pushed" by our doctors on behalf of their "suppliers", the pharmaceutical companies, but I'd much rather prescribe you an antidote myself! Here it is, the PaleoJay prescription for a long, healthy, happy, productive and disease free life:

1. Live a natural, ancestral type of lifestyle! Eat real foods, foods made by God and nature. Paleolithic foods, including

real organic veggies and fruits, wild caught meats and seafood, pastured butter and pork and cream and beef. Real oils like coconut oil and lard, beef tallow and olive oil.

2. Avoid modern wheat, which is modified in a lab and loaded with gluten, and most sugar. Sweeten slightly with local wild honey or maple syrup. Avoid processed foods, any kind of soda pop, and artificial sweeteners of any kind. And stay far from fast foods!

3. Avoid drugs, legal or illegal- the difference between them is not really that great!

4. Get at least 8 hours of good quality sleep, each and every night! Live with a connected "tribe" of people, relatives and friends, who try to get along and help one another and just connect as people are have evolved to do!

5. Avoid the medical system as much as you can, as often as you can! (To paraphrase John Wesley of Methodism fame). By this I mean, if you get in a car wreck or are shot with a bullet, our medical system is great at emergency types of medicine!

They can "patch you up" really well! But then, you need to get OUT of there as fast as you can, and start back in on steps 1-4 above- that is the only way to rebuild your health. The hospital knows nothing about rebuilding health, proper nutrition and lifestyle, or healthy movement and exercise! If you need to take a drug (like an antibiotic), take it and then STOP as soon as possible, and set about rebuilding your gut biome, which is all the friendly bacteria inside you that makes you healthy and happy- they are crucial, and if you take a course of antibiotics they are gone, right along with the unfriendly ones. Eat pre- and probiotics, kimchi and

sauerkraut, kefir and pickles, all must be naturally fermented!
Apple cider vinegar like Bragg's is one of the best sources of probiotics as well.

And as long as you are feeling well and healthy? STAY AWAY from organized medicine! Think of your local clinic as an old time medicine man, traveling from town to town with their "miracle elixir that cures everything"- they only want your money! Their elixir might not just be whisky and water like back in the old days, it might be a far slicker sales pitch, but the bottom line is the same:

They only want your money! Long ago, they only asked for a small amount for one bottle... but now they are so sophisticated about it they want eventually to take everything you have saved over a lifetime as they guide you out of this life!

Check out modern medical bills on life threatening surgeries and you'll see I'm right, especially in America!

The American average price was highest for every procedure but one.

Appendectomy
Average price in America: $13,910
Average price in Switzerland: $9,845
Average price in Argentina: $1,723
As with most procedures, there is a huge range in price even within the U.S. America's 25th percentile for appendectomies is $8,244, while the 95th percentile is $29,499. The Netherlands, Australia, and New Zealand are in the $5,000 range on average.
Normal delivery
Average price in America: $10,002

155

Average price in Switzerland: $8,307

Average price in Argentina: $2,237

The 95th percentile in the U.S. is a whopping $17,354 for a normal delivery. In Australia, the average is $6,623, in the Netherlands it's $2,824, and in Spain, $2,251. The American way of handling childbirth has been called the costliest in the world.

C-section

Average price in America: $15,240

Average price in Switzerland: $10,681

Average price in Spain: $2,844

In the U.S., the 95th percentile is $27,446 for a C-section. Switzerland and Australia are in the $10,000 range on average, while America's average is over $15,000. Argentina and Spain again had the lowest average prices, with the Netherlands falling in the middle at $5,492.

Cataract surgery

Average price in America: $3,762

Average price in Australia: $3,841

Average price in Argentina: $1,038

Only Australia shows one instance of a higher average price than the U.S., with cataract surgery costing just $79 more. The American 95th percentile is $8,233, showing just how much prices can vary. Even the 25th percentile, $2,422, is higher than the average prices in Argentina, the Netherlands, and Spain.

Knee replacement

Average price in America: $25,398

Average price in Switzerland: $24,614

Average price in Argentina: $6,015

The average price of a knee replacement is above $20,000 in New Zealand, Australia, and Switzerland, as well as the U.S. However, America's 95th percentile shoots up to $51,128. That's the cost of nearly nine knee replacements in Argentina.

Hip replacement

Average price in America: $26,489

Average price in Australia: $26,297

Average price in Argentina: $6,862

Hip replacements in Argentina, Spain, and the Netherlands all fall somewhere below $12,000 on average, yet America's 25th percentile for a hip replacement is $16,622, and the 95th percentile is $53,644. Artificial joint implants prices in the U.S. are inflated to begin with by the few companies that manufacture them, and then these prices are marked up several times by intermediaries, making artificial implants the single biggest cost of most joint replacement surgeries.

Bypass surgery

Average price in America: $75,345

Average price in Australia: $42,130

Average price in the Netherlands: $15,742

For bypass surgery, even America's 25th percentile of $47,982 is significantly higher than the average price of every other country surveyed. The figures for the Netherlands, Spain, and Argentina all fell under $17,000. The 95th percentile for a bypass surgery in America is $151,886.

Angioplasty

Average price in America: $27,907

Average price in New Zealand: $16,415

Average price in Argentina: $5,246

America's 25th and 95th percentiles for angioplasty show a wide range of $16,406 to $61,184. Average prices in Spain and Switzerland are in the $10,000 range, and Argentina, the Netherlands, and Switzerland boast even lower prices for this minimally invasive procedure.

Hip prosthesis

Average price in America: $11,806

Average price in Australia: $9,982

Average price in Spain: $3,177

Though Spain has the lowest figure by far, in New Zealand the average price of a hip prosthesis is $6,723, just over half the average U.S. price. With $25,843 as the 95th percentile, this procedure could conceivably be eight times more expensive when performed in the U.S. than it would be in Spain.

Buyer Beware! And best of all is to try to AVOID needing such surgeries by living an ancestral, paleo type of lifestyle!!

#

WOULD YOU GET A COLONOSCOPY FROM A USED CAR SALESMAN?

Here we go, another inflammatory diatribe by PaleoJay!
 Well, actually I don't think it really is, it's just contradicting another piece of "common medical wisdom and advice" that actually is quite dangerous, expensive, and health damaging.

It's this last that really bugs me, since medical care should above all obey the dictum to first do no harm. The inevitable harm caused by doing a full colonoscopy is the complete devastation of the gut biome, in other words all the little microbes that live in our guts and do things like control our body weight, mood, and the countless other vital processes we have not come close to mapping out yet.

Just like statin drug prescriptions, the colonoscopy seems to have become all about the money... at 5-10,000 dollars per scan, this is a huge moneymaker for medical clinics- why would they eliminate that cash cow for a little blood or stool test that costs a few hundred at most?

Well, the main reason would be because the blood or stool test is just as or MORE effective at detecting cancer, and there is no destruction of our precious gut biome, and no risk of perforation of the colon by the procedure, which is a very real danger! Why would you go into the hospital perfectly healthy, just to put yourself in extreme danger of being damaged, and with a certainty of making your health immediately worse, and your immune system compromised? It just doesn't make sense.

Just going under anesthesia is a real danger to you as well! And, it costs a lot of money too!

You can get a FOBT, a fecal occult blood test, a fecal immunochemical test, and the newest is called Cologuard.

Cologuard costs $599, which is a far cry from a colonoscopy. This is the kind of thing that really gets me doubting the motivations of our medical clinics, doctors, and system- they recommend things like colonoscopies that are expensive and dangerous with very little upside, and things like statin drugs for high cholesterol when there is no evidence that the symptom of high cholesterol really even causes heart disease, and they recommend multiple servings of grains per day to diabetes patients, and then sell them lots of insulin to mask the problems caused by the grains...

I could go on and on- but the obvious point is this:

IT'S ALL ABOUT THE MONEY!
IT'S NOT ABOUT YOUR HEALTH-
IT'S ALL ABOUT THE MONEY!

If you can be sick, and they sell you things to just treat the symptoms of that disease forever, wow- that's the best business model for them ever! There is absolutely no incentive to cure you of the disease, or of your many diseases.

Buyer beware. Don't ever go to the doctor and just do

whatever he or she says! Would you go to buy a new car and just buy whatever the salesman told you to? No, you'd do your research, look up the cars that interested you on the internet, compare prices and reviews, and then make your best decision based on knowledge.

Do the same thing with your health, but put in MORE time and research, because this is your HEALTH you are researching here. And it hurts me to say this, but try to imagine your doctor as a kind of seedy used car salesman, because that is what the profession has been tending towards in recent years. You don't have to say it, but keep it in the back of your mind.

And, if he tells you no, you can't screen for colon cancer with a blood test, tell him he's fired, and go to another doctor or clinic. You're the boss!

#

POLYPHARMACY AND DEATH BY DOCTOR

Polypharmacy is the use of four or more medications by a patient, generally adults aged over 65 years. Polypharmacy is most common in the elderly, affecting about 40% of older adults living in their own homes.

It is hard to believe that we have come to this, as a society!

Older adults, in particular, are more susceptible to this, since as a rule they have more medical conditions, and also they are from a time when people just "did what the Doctor said, no questions asked!" Let's hope that time is now GONE, at least for those of you listening to or reading these words!

Iatrogenesis is the word that means "Death by Doctor". This

160

means that if you follow a doctors advice and suggested treatment, that it winds up KILLING you! Rare, you think? Once in a blue moon??

Think again: Death by Doctor is now the third leading cause of death in America, right behind heart disease and cancer!

Some of these deaths are from botched surgeries, and infections picked up in the incredibly dangerous hospital environment...

But the vast majority are from prescribed medications, being taken as prescribed. The side effects of the medications, particularly in relation to one another, are that deadly!
We used to think of medicines as cure-alls- a simple PILL that would cure all our ILLS. We rarely consider that ALL pharmaceuticals have side effects, often side effects that are far worse than the disease or condition they are supposed to "cure". And they do not cure the condition! This is a common misconception: the vast majority of prescribed drugs just treat the symptoms, and do nothing to achieve a cure- only your own body, given enough healthy nutrients from good food, ample sleep, rest, and sunlight can cure itself.

Increasingly, our ever more potent and dangerous pharmaceuticals pose a real threat to our physical and mental health.

My own advice? Steer clear of modern medicine, as much as you can! You can do this by living a healthy lifestyle, eating right, ditching grains and sugars and loading up on green veggies, grass fed meats and dairy. Have a daily Green Smoothie, so you don't need a "drug cocktail" each day as you get older.
Invest in a Vitamix, so you don't have to buy an insulin pump

later.

And if you do have a medical condition already? Keep your medication list down to TWO at the most at any one time!

 Even with two medicines, the complications of side effects are staggering to monitor- get it down to ONE.

And I mean non-prescription drugs as well- Tylenol, Ibuprofen, even aspirin- these are toxic drugs, and also interact with other drugs in negative ways.

Even ONE modern, super potent, mind-altering drug is way more than a human should ever have to endure, but at least it can be isolated in its effects that way. I like to think of modern pharmaceutical medicines as similar to modern processed fake "foods" like fast food, breakfast cereals, and pop tarts- horrible JUNK that should be completely avoided as much as possible!

The human population used to live long, healthy lives with no drugs. Once a person survived childbirth, they lived just as long (or longer!) than modern Americans do today. Go into any old cemetery and read the born and died dates. The only thing that makes people think we all live longer today is because we have eliminated almost all of the deaths in childbirth of both mothers and children. That skews the statistics in favor of modern lifespans.

But, the quality of life is also very different- heart disease, cancer, diabetes- virtually all the diseases of modern life we now take for granted hardly even existed back then! And let's not forget one of the biggest modern killers of all- iatrogenesis, or death by doctor!

#

GORGE YOURSELF ON THE GOOD

I was at a 60th birthday party recently- (I am 63 myself), and was surprised to find that a party is, at this point in life, often a place to talk about... illness.

Illnesses and the DRUGS to treat them!

I had this strange feeling that I was a seer: I knew what each person talking really needed, a bit of information that would rectify what was wrong with them; would save them, if you will, from disease, disability, and eventual premature death!

The only problem is that... I really can't say anything!

This is what a knowledge of the Ancestral way of living does to you! You know what almost everyone needs to restore their health- get rid of their degenerative diseases, that are gradually destroying their health, wellness, and quality of life...

But you also know that they don't want to hear it!

You're not a Doctor! You're not qualified!

But, most importantly: they don't want to change their habits- their way of eating and living! NO NO NO!

It's ironic, but Medical Doctors know nothing about nutrition- nothing! In fact, they as a rule tend to discount its importance entirely.

It's really crazy that someone like PaleoJay, a 63 year old English major in college, knows more than an MD from Harvard or anywhere else-
but it's TRUE!

163

Just as someone like Jimi Hendrix learned through actually doing it how to express himself musically through a guitar - so it is that if you endeavor to educate yourself about your own health and wellness by actually doing, and exploring ideas and experimenting rather than just following accepted rote dogma- you can actually fix your own health!

And that of others, like your family and friends, if they do choose to listen.

Back to before: virtually EVERYONE, by the age of 60, has LOTS of medical issues- metabolic syndrome, diabesity, skin conditions, actual diabetes itself, obesity and heart disease, chronic stress and high blood pressure; difficulty sleeping, rheumatoid arthritis, even cancer...

The incredible secret I want to tell you here is that:

ALL OF THESE ARE PREVENTABLE, AND EVEN REVERSIBLE!

Right now, I'm not at a party with friends- I'm here, talking to YOU, my BEST friend! And I'm here to tell you that if you just EAT real, God made foods; foods like grass fed meat, pastured eggs, LOTS of veggies (especially whipped up in a Vitamix blender/smoothie!), pastured dairy like butter and cream- preferably raw!, get LOTS of sleep, rest and recreation- do SOME bodyweight and virtually resistance exercises most days- walk as much as you can daily, spend time with friends and family on a regular basis (not just watching tv together), and get out in the SUN for at least 15 minutes per day, preferably in a natural, forest or savvanah-like environment...

YOU SHOULN'T NEED ANY PHARMACEUTICAL

MEDICINES AT ALL- EVER!!

Of course, if you also eliminate BREAD, and pasta, and anything containing gluten whatsoever, like... almost everything that is manmade like fast food, deli food, breakfast food, sandwich food, food food- in other words- MAN MADE PROCESSED FOODS-

YOU WILL BE GOLDEN!!

BUT, I think that most people getting into the Ancestral lifestyle concentrate on ELIMINATING foods; which is why I concentrate on ADDING IN nutrient dense, good, GOD MADE FOODS!

If you do that: you won't want, or have room for the man made CRAP.

And so, concentrate on adding in as much as you possibly can of good, wholesome God made foods!

To paraphrase John Wesley:

Eat as much God made food as you can!
As often as you can! With all the friends that you can! With all the people that you can! As long as ever you can!

Sorry to go all evangelical on you, but I feel that strongly about this.

The more of good food you eat, the less of the bad!

Gorge yourself on the GOOD

In SLEEP, in family and friend relations- at church, and with your neighbors!

165

PaleoJay's Smoothie Cafe!

GORGE yourself on a daily exercise regimen in the early morning doing Perfectly Paleo Exercise- POUR Veggie and Vitamin rich smoothie into your body morning and noon... FAST at night, regulating your body in tune with it's ancestral rhythms of feast and famine- sing and dance with your friends- have campfires and wander through the forest, getting in tune with nature!! Go to bed EARLY, and wake up EARLY- get in touch with your circadian rhythms!

And now? Life is good! Who even WANTS a donut?
#

YOU ARE YOUR OWN DOCTOR

It's true- YOU are your own doctor- your own healer! Especially in today's world, with the internet, there is absolutely no excuse for YOU not be in total touch with your own health challenges.

You have the internet waiting and ready to answer questions about your health problems- you have podcasts like PaleoJay's Smoothie Cafe, Paleo Quick Tip of the Day, and many others as well to answer your questions, give you insights as to the how and why of the ancestral lifestyle- Blogs like www.paleojay.com, www.mark'sdailyapple.com, robbwolf.com, www.livinlavidalowcarb.com, thepaleodiet.com, and many others- take advantage of these!

Podcasts are ideal, because you can do other things while you learn and are entertained all at once- things like driving could be a time sink; but, fill them with podcasts of value, and you are going to the university while you drive! Same with mowing, washing dishes, chores- it makes it fun and very, very profitable for your health at the same time! My favorite app for podcasts is Downcast- the free Podcast app from Apple is fine, and so is Stitcher. Hey- give me a recommendation on iTunes or Stitcher, and it will really help other people to find me, and let me help them, like I am hopefully helping YOU. Paleo is starting to take over on the health front, and rightfully so, because it is the real deal- it works- not just for a month, or a year, or five years- FOR A LIFETIME IT WORKS!

You are on the cusp of a revolution my friend. Doesn't it feel great to be a Paleo Pioneer?? A role model for your friends and family? Well, if you are "going Paleo"- YOU ARE!

You are also, as I said above: Your own Doctor!

If you go to a medical doctor, realize that he is just a hired consultant; nothing more. DOCTOR doesn't even MEAN healer- it means teacher.

And modern medical Doctors can only teach you about disease- and they can only treat the symptoms, not the causes of most modern degenerative diseases that are destroying our health in the modern world- and they can only treat these symptoms with drugs, drugs that are LOADED with bad side-effects- side effects that are often worse than the disease itself.

So, take charge. Be your own doctor! How? Well, grasshopper:

Eat an ancestral diet. Eliminate grains- they have very little nutrition anyway; especially whole grains! Whole grains, of wheat, brown rice, wild rice, are loaded with anti-nutrients, i.e. POISONS designed to keep mammals like US from eating them. They are also by and large purely sugar in terms of our glycemic response and triggering an insulin surge- avoid them.

PaleoJay's Smoothie Cafe!

Eat grass fed meat, pastured dairy- especially fatty dairy like cream, butter, full fat Greek yogurt, kefir.

LOTS of seafood like sardines, wild caught salmon and other fish as well, shrimp, oysters and anchovies.

TONS of veggies! This is the hardest part- our ancestors basically chewed on vegetables ALL DAY LONG whenever they could- the varieties available in the past were small and tough, but our ancestors knew their importance in health and survival. The best way to get them into your diet in abundance in the modern world is to VITAMIX them into a smoothie each and every day! Easy, effective, convenient, and the very healthiest thing you can do for you and your family, bar none- get a Vitamix! Make Paleo Smoothies!

And, this may surprise you, but eat WHITE RICE, white potato (NO SKIN!), and sweet potatoes... originally most Paleo gurus were ultra-low carb, and anti-potato, but nowadays the consensus for most is that including 15-30% of these SAFE STARCHES into your diet is not only not bad, but very beneficial to your health! This is still far less carbs, and WAY safer carbs than are consumed on the SAD diet; but these safe starches also keep down fungus in your system which is encouraged by either a very LOW or a very HIGH carb diet. Also, resistant starches that you do not digest yourself when you consume them, like reheated rice and white potato feed your gut microbes instead, which is VERY beneficial to your health indeed- our gut microbes do incredible things in terms of regulating our mood, sleep, and overall health and digestion.

One more tip is to eat LESS OFTEN. Try to fast, or not eat for about 16 hours or so most days- this allows for autophagy, which is a term for "routine maintenance" of your body, by your body!

168

PaleoJay's Smoothie Cafe!

If you are constantly digesting, your poor body can't take care of "little things" like killing cancer cells, consuming damaged mitochondria, and otherwise doing housekeeping of your bodies cells to keep them healthy and vital! A short break from eating, which is natural, and what our bodies expect and have been made to take advantage of is one of the most healthy, and life-extending things we can do...

So, skip either breakfast like most paleo people do; or supper, like me!

 I like to have a BIG Paleo breakfast, with eggs, and salsa, and a big Paleo Smoothie, and pastured bacon and/or sausage most mornings...

A big, giant salad topped with meat or seafood, or heated pastured beef or pork or shrimp and veggies atop some reheated white rice for lunch, and then ANOTHER big Paleo Smoothie late afternoon- and then I'm DONE!
Stuffed and happy- ready to be busy, or relax, read, or play music, or whatever I want with friends and family until an early bedtime...

OR, on days off I often take the standard Intermittent fasting approach and Skip Breakfast; having coffee with a little coconut oil in it, topped with whipped cream, cinnamon and cloves (usually while I exercise in the living room in front of the TV doing Perfectly Paleo Exercise), and don't eat until maybe 11 or 12:00... either way works, and really frees up time to do productive things rather than just EATING! It's kind of like autophagy for your life as well as for your body- by not digesting, your body gets a break, and by not having to prepare, eat, and clean up YOU get a break!
Win Win!

So, that is how to build up your bodies TERRAIN- your natural health, so that your own immune system can keep you healthy, and disease free!

A healthy terrain, or body, means that you won't need a doctor, or anyone else, to restore your health, since you are doing it yourself, naturally, like humans have done for thousands and thousands of years, successfully! It's all about good, nutritious, healthy God made food, LOTS of sleep, lots of God made vegetables and rice and potatoes, lots of animal protein and collagen and fats as provided for us by God (remember the Fatted Calf!)-

And staying active, and flexible, and strong, and vital and lean by doing our Perfectly Paleo Exercises on a daily basis, pleasurably and naturally, whilst sipping our coffee or green or white tea, loaded with anti-oxidants, and enjoying the early morning air in our lungs while we watch a great Netflix movie- reveling in the fact that we have a healthy TERRAIN- we are very, very healthy indeed, and have no need of a symptoms treating MD at all...

Since we have become our own doctor!

#

BE A PALEO ROLE MODEL

It won't be long until eating a paleo diet will be like not smoking cigarettes! I know, it sounds far fetched in these benighted times, when if you order a burger without a bun gets you incredulous looks from all around you, but give it time, my friends...

If you are in my age group you will realize just how much cigarette smoking was ingrained in the American culture of not that long ago (the 1960's). I am 63 now, and remember well the day of extensive cigarette ads on TV and radio, the vending machines on every corner that sold cigarette packs to anyone with 35 cents, and how every home had multiple ash trays set around inside... even in households that did not contain a smoker!

When I was a child, even though neither of my parents smoked, most of their friends did, and so it was my job to empty the ash trays after they visited! Actually, if anything will put you off of cigarette smoking, it would be that job of emptying the leftover ashes and especially those icky lipstick smeared butts...

It was mainly a "cultural thing" back then, and I believe that eating wheat products like altered, modern bread and cereals will look just like cigarette smoking in the future! The science is all there, backing up the health benefits of ditching grains and sugars- it just hasn't filtered out into the mainstream as of yet!

What do you think, and how do you react when you see a pregnant woman drinking alcohol? Or nursing her baby (well, in this case she'd probably use formula instead) while smoking a cigarette??

You recoil in horror, right?

Wait a few years, and when you see a mother giving her little children a happy meal of crappy fake hamburger meat on a huge bun with fries and a coke, you will recoil just the same!

It will NOT be socially acceptable any longer, and rightfully so.

It will still be with us, since we are a free country, thankfully...but there will be strong disapproval from all about it.

The time will come when your fellow workers will not be proud of eating a candy bar, and guzzling a mountain dew for breakfast in the morning, since they stayed up too late and didn't get enough sleep...

They will be ashamed. Again, and rightfully so- the information will have filtered down to the masses- everyone who has a brain, at least, will get it-

Sugar, and grains are BAD! Vegetables, natural fats and meats are wonderful, and above all- OUR HEALTH IS UP TO US!

Conventional medicine only masks symptoms; it does not cure the cause- that is up to us, our own diet and lifestyle choices!

And, when everyone finally knows that, why then anyone who does not make the right choices might as well be wearing a dunce cap and a clown nose.

THEY WILL LOOK LIKE AN IDIOT!!

So, go ahead and look like a genius, way ahead of your time.

Make a green smoothie, and drink it daily. Eat grass fed meat and dairy, pastured eggs and dairy, tons of veggies, and become your OWN doctor- avoid pharmaceutical medicines as much as you can! They cause more deaths by far than illegal drugs!!
Sleep 8 hours each night, and exercise with natural Perfectly Paleo types of body weight exercises each day. Develop a good tribe of family and friends!

* * *

PaleoJay's Smoothie Cafe!

You will be healthy and happy, but even more importantly:
YOU WILL BE A ROLE MODEL FOR THE FUTURE!

Skin and Dental Health!

SAVE YOUR TEETH AND SKIN NATURALLY- WITH COCONUT

Coconut oil is so good for you, internally, that to go for even a day without ingesting at least some coconut oil seems terrible to me- kind of like the old "a day without sunshine" quote! I mean, talk about a good, God made type of fat- one that nourishes every cell in your body by supplying them with lauric acid, for instance.

Lauric acid can help lower your cholesterol and blood pressure, keeps your arteries flexible and atherosclerosis free.

Coconut oil is also a metabolism booster- I know when I first started adding coconut milk and oil to my Paleo smoothie, I immediately lost over 5 pounds I didn't even know I had to lose- really! It was all visceral fat, meaning around my internal organs, so it really didn't show, but that is the most dangerous kind of fat for your health. Thanks, coconut oil!

But, did you know that the external benefits of coconut oil are just as profound?

I always recommend having a jar of good, expeller pressed coconut oil in both the kitchen- and the bathroom. The one in the bathroom is a skin lotion par exellance! If you whip it with a blender, and maybe put in a few drops of an herbal oil like peppermint or lavender, it will be airy,light and creamy-

just put some on your hands when you get out of the shower, and coat your skin from face down to your toes! NOTHING is better for your skin than this natural, coconut oil cream...AND the lauric acid and many other beneficial components of the oil will absorb into your bloodstream, right through your skin! (Makes you kind of leery of petroleum, chemical based skin lotions, doesn't it? It should- THEY are absorbed through your skin in the same way.)

Also, to shave with coconut oil is the best lubricant you can find- healthy and moisturizing, without feeling greasy in the slightest. And, you can and should just leave the remainder on after shaving- men and women both! Coconut oil is both antifungal, and antibacterial...

It's also great as a hair conditioner- just rub it into your hair and scalp, and leave in for a few hours, then shampoo. Your hair will be soft, moisturized, and revitalized!

What about the TEETH? Well, the antibacterial effect of a mouthful of coconut oil is amazing, not to mention that it de-acidifies your mouth, teeth and gums- this acidity is what really harms our teeth, encouraging the growth of harmful bacteria that erode our teeth and gums. You can even brush your teeth with coconut oil... but, the very best thing you can do for your oral health period- I believe this even is more important than brushing or flossing- is coconut oil pulling!

Just take about a teaspoonful before you shower, and put it in your mouth. Swish it around, or "pull" it through your teeth and around your mouth for the length of your shower, and shaving, and the rest of your morning routine- then, last thing before you leave the bathroom to get dressed- spit out the oil into the toilet.

* * *

175

That oil you just spit out is holding all of the bacteria, acidity, and just plain pollution that has accumulated inside your mouth. So now, you mouth, teeth, gums and entire oral cavity are rejuvenated, pristine, and on the way to perfect health.

And if you then take some more coconut oil in by way of your daily Paleo Smoothie, so is the rest of you on that same journey!

#

PALEO DIET FOR HEALTHY SKIN, HAIR, AND TEETH

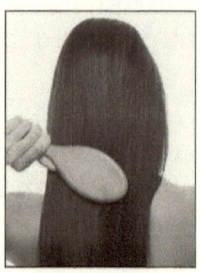

I know, you want to eat a paleo type of diet because it will make you leaner, stronger, and fitter; meaning you are more defined, can lift heavier things, and have more endurance to do just about anything... but have you thought about the ancillary things about living within the Paleolithic template, or ancestral diet that are just as important, but you haven't heard about?

One of the most fast and remarkable changes brought about by adopting the Paleo diet is greatly improved skin health!

By eliminating the phytates, the anti-nutrients that are within grains, particularly wheat, inflammation is drastically reduced!

Inflammation is the root cause of most modern disease, but it is also the cause of skin problems- acne, rosacea, psoriasis; even simple things like dry skin, or oily skin...

Your body starts to just work like it should,because it has the nutrients (or the building blocks) from which to work properly! And, it has not been "gummed up" with all of the worthless crap from industrial seed oils, loads and loads of sugars and artificial sweeteners, margarines- you get the picture- it's just as if you put all of this stuff into your car's gas tank- do you think it would run well? Or even at all after a short time!

The same thing is true of your dental health- in my opinion, it would be well worth embracing the paleo diet just for the benefits to your teeth and gums alone! The results are that dramatic. After the first few months of adopting the paleo diet, years ago,my wife and I both had checkups at our long-time dentist. We had good checkups, as always, but the hygienist was amazed- what had we been doing? There was virtually NO plaque or tartar buildup, and our gums were just pristine! She seemed genuinely flabbergasted. All we had done was eliminate wheat, at that point, and begun our daily Paleo

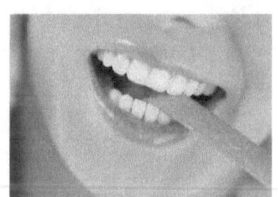

Hair health is similar- I guarantee your hair will feel thicker, and will definitely be much shinier after starting to include plenty of healthy fats, like pastured butter and coconut oil!

And without the grains in the way, and displacing the eating of other really nutrient dense foods like grass fed meat, seafood, and those good fats, the body can really go to town putting nutrients to work in "non-essential" areas- like the skin, teeth, hair, and even the eyes! If you eat a nutrient poor diet, like most modern Americans do today, the body is forced to "triage" the nutrients it has, using them to perform vital functions of survival, like keeping the organs working, the heart beating, and the brain functioning, at least at a low level...

If the nutrients are all present and accounted for, and ABUNDANT, the body has the luxury of working on those "non-essential" parts of us that we care so much about- it can give us glowing, healthy skin!

It can give us shiny, abundant hair! It can put the High lutein and zeaxanthin pigments that are found in eggs, and green leafy veggies to good work, repairing our vision!
The teeth can, and WILL REMINERALIZE themselves, if only we give them the raw materials, and the minerals they need through our diet! Even cavities can remineralize and heal- Whole Grains INHIBIT the ability to digest minerals!

Isn't this the type of results that you are interested in? Isn't EVERYONE? Save your vision, your teeth... have healthy skin and hair... and incidentally be disease free, full of energy, and have a healthy, well functioning mind and body- eat a Paleo type of diet!

* * *

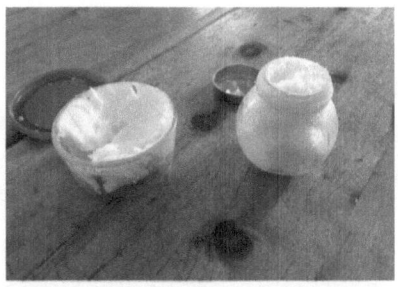

Get a big jar of organic, virgin coconut oil- in fact, get TWO-
one for the bathroom, one for the kitchen! The bathroom
coconut oil is perfect to rub on your skin after your shower-
it is not only the BEST moisturizer you can find, it is also a
great anti-bacterial AND a mild sunscreen. Mild is what you
want, since you DO want vitamin D to be synthesized from
the sun- and it is chemical free!

Once you get yourself a Vitamix, and make a daily green
paleo smoothie, you will save yourself a lot of time, since you
make the smoothie in the morning, and it pretty much gives
you all the nutrients you could possibly need for the day, in a
quickly made, drinkable form that you can carry with you-
and all made from REAL FOODS!

So, picture yourself and your family, glowing with health, at
your ideal weight, all just two things:
Eliminating BAD, FAKE foods like wheat, tons of sugar and
artificial sweeteners, and industrial seed oils, and
Adding in tons of REAL foods, like grass fed meats, coconut
oil and pastured butter, seafood, fruits and veggies!

Throw in 8 hours of quality sleep per night, a bit of visualized
resistance, Perfectly Paleo Exercise on a frequent basis, and
you will be so healthy, both mentally AND physically, that
your life, and that of your family, will be TRANSFORMED!
It really is that easy!

#

GETTING RID OF EYEGLASSES

I wore eyeglasses from my teens, until I was in my late 50's...

I never really thought about it much, except that it was kind of a pain. Especially when exercising, skiing, playing sports- come to think about it, it kind of got in the way in almost everything I loved doing! Except for maybe reading...

And, my prescription got stronger every time I went in for a checkup! I never thought about it, but my eyes were steadily getting weaker, year after year, even while my progressively strength trained body got stronger. It was only when I found out about the supreme importance of nutrition, specifically the paleo diet of real food- meat, seafood, vegetables, healthy fats, nuts seeds and fruits- that is when my health took a dramatic turn for the better!

But this is about eyesight, right?

The truth about minus lenses: (Minus lenses are those that make objects appear closer, in other words if your are nearsighted).
Minus lenses create the need for stronger glasses YEAR AFTER YEAR!
Minus lenses cause the eye to lengthen ABNORMALLY!
Minus lenses greatly increase the risk of RETINAL DETACHMENT, CATARACT and RETINOPATHY!
Minus lenses cause myopia that doctors treat with RISKY CORNEAL SURGERY!
Minus lenses are a crutch that must be worn a LIFETIME!
Minus lenses lead to eye exams and corrective lenses that are EXPENSIVE!
Minus lenses enrich the eye doctors and destroy YOUR

180

HEALTH!

Minus lenses and their frames reduce peripheral vision and are HAZARDOUS!

Minus lenses have never been proven SAFE!

Minus lenses can lead to BLINDNESS!

Minus lenses and the doctors who recommend them are your ENEMIES

But, for now, just remember this- eyeglasses are casts for your eyes!

If you wear a cast on your arm, what happens? That's right, the arm in the cast withers, and weakens- and quite quickly and dramatically, too!!

Wear these "casts" on your eyes, year after year, and what can you expect but dramatic decrease in eye sight strength? How can you avoid this?

First off- don't get stronger prescriptions! Insist on a slightly weaker prescription, if you are already wearing glasses. Get one just strong enough that you can, with some effort, make out what you are looking at. Do this, and the next time you go to the Eye Dr., get an even weaker prescription.

I know this sounds strange, but let me say this: I no longer wear glasses at all, and this is after over 40 years of wearing them! I can't tell you how liberating it feels, in more ways than just improved eyesight!

One of the major benefits I have noticed is that, since my left eye was considerably weaker than my right eye, and the right, intuitive side of the brain controls the left eye, my creative side was stifled and controlled by the left, dogmatic, purely logical side of my brain!

* * *

181

Now that my left eye is stronger than my right, it has wrought a profound personality "shift", making me a much more creative, free-thinking, live-in-the-moment kind of person.

Also, I believe that just the constant act of looking at life through little lenses puts you in the position of being "removed" from the action- makes you more of an "observer" than as a real, living, participant in life!

Leaving glasses behind is really that life changing!

OK, so how do you do it? Simple- just don't wear glasses when you don't need them! (First step)

It depends how bad your vision has deteriorated, but many of us really don't need glasses as soon as we get up, to walk to the bathroom- yet we often put them on immediately! Don't! If you can read without glasses, don't put them on! If you need them currently to drive, take them off when you get there!

When you read, move the print back just enough that you can make out the print. Don't make it too easy- make your eyes work- and periodically look up, and focus on something farther away. If you are far sighted, do the opposite! Move the print closer; make your eyes focus just "on the edge" of where it starts to go out of focus.

You get the idea! Gradual eye improvement will happen, if you let it, naturally! Just minimize the unnatural times you immobilize your eyes behind the casts of eyeglasses or contact lenses!

One other thing I'm convinced of is that, just as in all else in health, eating a paleo, or ancestral diet, consisting of REAL

FOODS and devoid of grains, sugars, and industrial seed oils if paramount in restoring and building the health of your eyesight, or of any other part of your body or your mind!

Nutrition can make or break anything you do- it really is that important!!

Work at your vision, and you may, like me, surprise yourself and become free of glasses!

Here is another excellent link: www.pinholeglasses.com

Just be persistent, and get in touch with an optometrist that works in Behavioral Optometry!

Other optometrists tend to be...resistant to working with your desire to lessen your prescription. Just as most standard MD's tend to be resistant to the idea of "Letting nutrition be thy medicine, and medicine be thy food", despite the fact that that last is a quote from Hippocrates, the founder of Western Medicine, whom all Medical Doctors are sworn to follow! Ironic, I know, but there are good and bad doctors, just like there are good and bad in all walks of life...

#

BETTER LIVING withOUT CHEMISTRY!

One thing that I have noticed that many Paleo People seem to omit from the many changes they make in implementing an ancestral or paleo type of lifestyle is to eliminate some really bad things. They give up grains (hard) and minimize sugars (also hard to do) in their lives, take up daily exercise and easy movement, and go to bed early to get a full 8 hours plus of sleep per night in a totally blacked-out bedroom.
 They take great pains to cultivate their tribe of family, friends and church, connecting and inter-reacting on a regular basis! They are almost THERE...

183

But they still go to the store, and buy incredibly toxic products, products of poison like chemical cleaners, personal care products like soaps and shampoos that are loaded with petroleum byproducts like sodium lauryl sulphate. Sulfates strip the skin of its natural oils and increase penetration of the skin's surface. They are also irritants for people with sensitive skin or eczema. This is in almost every commercial soap or body wash and shampoo, and eliminating it made a huge difference for me!

Fragrance. Bottom line: If the ingredient is vague, it's probably hiding something. "Fragrance" could actually be a cocktail of chemicals and you'd never know it. The FDA doesn't require companies to disclose the breakdown of a fragrance's ingredients to consumers because the chemicals that produce fragrance are considered "trade secrets." Most of the time, synthetic chemicals and cancer-causing toxins (like phthalates, used to make fragrances last longer) are hiding under that one sneaky term. Constant exposure to fragrances has been shown to negatively impact the central nervous system and can trigger allergies, migraines and asthma symptoms.

Parabens. These ingredients are estrogen mimickers— meaning that once applied to the skin, they enter the bloodstream, and the body mistakes them for estrogen. When the body thinks there is an abnormally high amount of estrogen present in the bloodstream due to the presence of these hormone disrupters, it reacts in various ways: decreasing muscle mass, increasing fat deposits, causing early onset of puberty and spurring reproductive difficulties in both men and women.

And lastly, there is Triclosan. This chemical is most often found in antibacterial soap. Recent studies have found that

184

triclosan actually promotes the emergence and growth of bacteria resistant to antibiotic cleansers. It also creates dioxin, a carcinogen that has been found in high levels in human breast milk. Dioxins have disruptive effects on theendocrine system and negatively affect thyroid functions. And here's a fun fact: dioxin is the primary toxic component of Agent Orange!

Think about it. If we are washing our bodies with soap that contains harmful ingredients every single day, this adds up over a lifetime to wreak havoc on our health.

Since there is minimal government testing on these chemicals, it becomes up to us, as smart consumers, to make informed decisions as to what does and doesn't go on our skin.

Get good quality, natural, coconut oil based or other natural fat based soaps, shampoos and body washes. They are out there: God made products, combined in low tech ways to make honest to God products!

Just like you should only eat natural, God made foods, you should only use natural, God made cleaning products...

And don't even THINK about throwing a little Roundup on those cracks in your sidewalk... oh my God- the main ingredient in roundup by Monsanto is glyphosate.

Glyphosate affects your gut bacteria just as it does weeds in your yard.

It causes extreme disruption of your beneficial microbes' functions and life cycles. This sets YOU up for autoimmune disease! By killing your beneficial bacteria, which it tends to do preferentially, it allows your BAD, sugar-thriving bacteria to multiply, causing things like small intestinal bacterial overgrowth, or SIBO, and all of the downstream results of fat weight gain, acid reflux, asthma, and- again- autoimmune diseases of all sorts.

Since this is paleo QUICK tip, I will stop there...

But, later, we should talk about the little shop of cosmetic horrors...

Essential Oils!

ESSENTIAL OILS ARE ESSENTIAL

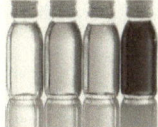

Something you are probably not doing along with your ancestral lifestyle of natural exercise and real, God made food diet is using natural medicines. I'm talking about essential oils, and if you don't know about them, or think they are some crazy hippy thing- well, they're not!

I would recommend you purchase some quality ones, and keep them in your medicine cabinet for naturally treating yourself and your family! Here are some of the very best to have on hand and use regularly:

Tea tree oil- this is a great antiseptic! I love it in my diffuser, which is a device that puts water vapor into the air mixed with essential oils. For me, this is the very best way to get the best of all that essential oil has to offer. You will never sleep better than when you put say, tea tree oil and peppermint essential oils together in your diffuser. Just put a few drops of one or more essential oil in the water in your diffuser- steam comes out slowly, infused with the oils scent and medicinal properties, and will lull you to sleep while getting the medicinal values of the oils into your body through your inhalations. And it smells great!

Lavender oil is another I recommend, along with lemon, frankincense, (pretend a wise man gave it to you)peppermint and oregano. There are other wonderful oils, but these are all a great place to start, and kind of cover all the bases.

Many oils help with mental states as well- lavender and lemon oils are "mood lifters" and can combat depression and even headaches. Peppermint is another disinfectant and antiseptic oil, and is wonderful for dental care. I currently brush my teeth with a combination of peppermint and tea tree oil- I believe that this, along with

#

RECOVERING FROM ILLNESS WITH ESSENTIAL OILS AND REST

As usual, I am writing this from my own personal experience coupled along with research. I awoke ill yesterday, on Wednesday, with a bad (and worsening) sore throat, and a deep cough settled down in my chest! I virtually never get sick, but it has been exceptionally cold here in Wisconsin, and I have been running around outside and inside stores, where I must have picked up a bug of some sort.

Yes, even Mr. PaleoJay is not immune to getting sick or injured- none of us are, no matter how much we improve our our bodily terrain or avoid bad situations. And so, it is important to know just what to do when we do get sick!

When I realized I was sick yesterday, I got up and went downstairs, and prepared a paleo green smoothie since the ball canning jars I had filled earlier in the week were used up. (I like to stock my fridge with a few days supply of the healthiest form of nutrition I can devise!)

Step 1 in recuperation: maximize nutrition, so the body can rebuild the damages and repair the defenses!

Next, I repaired to the living room with my smoothie and a cup of hot green tea in hand! Wrapping myself in a sleeping bag that I love to sit beneath on winter days, I turned on Netflix and streamed away on my latest show- Spartacus! I tried to stay as warm and relaxes as possible... then, remembering my essential oil diffuser, I went and got that, loaded it with water along with Frankincense and Lavender

189

oils, and set it right beside my easy chair, and again wrapped myself in my sleeping bag.

And that is how I spent my morning- Watching television, then dozing for awhile, then reading my iphone, then dozing... and so it went on...

If you know me at all, you know this is not my morning routine! Normally, every single morning I start with a workout, and then I get going on stuff- writing, reading, updating, researching! Walking, cooking, shoveling snow- just lots of movement and action. I thrive on the feeling of accomplishment, as I believe most of us do.

But not this sick morning- the best accomplishment I could achieve would be to get WELL!

And so, that is largely how my day went- with purposeful rest, only the best in nutrition (I had little appetite), and finally going back to bed again, at a very early hour. I set the diffuser with a fresh load of essential oils at my bedside, and went to sleep...

And by this morning, although the infection had resided deep in my chest, and I was developing a wracking cough at bedtime-

By the morning, after about 11 hours of off again, on again sleep-

My sickness had become a cold! And now, it is 4 PM of that day, Thursday, and what had threatened to take me down for at least a week has subsided into just a stuffed up nose.

But now, here it is today, only one day later, and I am largely sickness free-

* * *

Makes me feel like singing Everything is Awesome!

\#

COFFEE IS AN ESSENTIAL OIL

I know, this sounds crazy! But then again, don't most of my
ideas? (Don't answer that).

But truly: I get so tired over the years of criticisms of coffee!
 I think this is like criticisms of anything that people enjoy- it
must be bad, right? Well, in this case, wrong! To the
contrary, in our modern, neolithic, grain and sugar based
diet, coffee is for most people the major source of
antioxidants in their diet. This is kind of a shocker, but
nonetheless very true.
After all, for normal, non paleo kinds of folks, who only get
green veggies and colorful berries once in a blue moon, who
subsist on fast food hamburgers, pizza, and french fries-
coffee is IT- their only antioxidant! Sad but true...here is a
quote-
Coffee is a rich source of disease-fighting antioxidants. And
studies have shown that it may reduce cavities, boost athletic
performance, improve moods, and stop headaches -- not to
mention reduce the risk of type 2 diabetes, colon cancer, liver
cancer, gall stones, cirrhosis of the liver, and Parkinson's
diseases!

After you start to look into it, it is kind of startling all of the
great benefits of what has been painted as evil for so long-
but, then again, consider how FAT and red meat has likewise
been equated with evil for so long, and also how grains and
sugar have been given a complete angelic halo by the
mainstream medical establishment.

Well, now it starts to make sense, doesn't it?

191

PaleoJay's Smoothie Cafe!
* * *

Big Government agencies and mainstream medicine misled us about grains and sugar, fat and red meat for so long, why shouldn't we also be suspicious of their other "advice"!!??

Like coffee being bad for us. It's not, it never has been, and is actually quite beneficial in many ways.

How you brew it can make a difference, however- along with what you put in it! Here is what I do:

I make my coffee with an Aerobie Press! It is a plunger type of apparatus, and costs about $20 or so. I heat the water in an electric carafe or tea kettle, and pour it in my press, which fits into individual cups. Then, I just press it through one cup, then another, and then another! (Two for me, one for my loving, appreciative wife!)

Just get a good, organic coffee, and you are good to go! The rumours about "mold" in coffee are unfounded, unless you get cheap, supermarket type of generic coffees.... they are not a good choice, either for flavor or health! Get a good organic (I like French Roast), and grind it yourself for maximum flavor.

Now comes the best part- adding flavor (and additional healthiness!) to your coffee.

I always add about a teaspoon of good coconut oil to each cup.
This adds in a really healthy fat, that will fill you up, and also load you up with medium chain fatty acids, that are the most digestible, beneficial, and anti-bacterial and anti-inflammatory type of food you can consume!
Really!

* * *

PaleoJay's Smoothie Cafe!

Coconut oil is the best fat you can consume, and probably the best FOOD you can consume! Start each and every day with it, in your coffee, and you are halfway to health!!

Add in whipped or just plain full fat cream, cinnamon and cloves, perhaps some cacao powder as I do...

Then, open one of your 16 oz. Ball jars of Paleo Green Smoothie, loaded with veggies and berries and kefir and cod liver oil and.... well, look it up at www.paleojay.com perfectly paleo smoothie ingredients.

You now have breakfast, a wonderful coffee beverage to comfort you as you work out in front of the television with Perfectly Paleo Exercise, and an assurance that, not only are you starting your day in the healthiest way possible, but you won't be hungry for many hours!

You can easily make good food choices when you are not starving, but just interested in maximizing nutrition.
As they say, "Once begun, half done"!
So start your day in the perfectly paleo way, with coffee!!

Avoid Health Scams!

What's Wrong with Vaccinations?

There is a real problem in how the Federal Government, Big Pharmaceuticals, and Big Medicine have been handling the vaccinations in this country. Voices are shrill from those that are in power over US, the people in the U.S.- you MUST get vaccinated- if you don't you are endangering everyone! And so, the line of reasoning is tending in this direction- we will make you get them! Government Control!!

This is a major problem, since those big 3 organizations of Big Government, Big Pharma, and Big Medicine are mainly concerned with PROFIT, not our health. These are the same entities that have given us the Food Pyramid dominated by grains, sugar, and low fat everything. Under these guidelines, the American people have become more sick and inflamed than ever before!

More importantly even than the effects of all of this bad food, and poor lifestyle of endless sitting, little sleep, and no real nutrition is what this behavior does to our gut microbes- the tiny GOOD bacteria that we have co-evolved with, and that keep us healthy, improving the terrain of our bodies so that we can fight off BAD bacteria!

It's similar to what happened to dairy in this country when we allowed big dairy to industrialize away from small farms, and crowd cows together in filthy conditions with no access to good grass and space to move, and instead loaded them up with spent grains from the brewing industry in the early

194

1900's. Suddenly, milk needed to be pasteurized! Our cows were leading lives like most of us do today- not exercising properly, or sleeping, or getting out in nature as we are meant to, and being jammed all together in huge numbers- they were chronically sick animals, just as now we are all chronically sick.

Oh, and they also started to need huge amounts of antibiotics, and other medicines and vaccines just to survive long enough to slaughter... Sound familiar?

If we insist on living unhealthy, SAD types of lives, we will sadly have to take many medicines just to relieve the symptoms of diabesity and all related modern illnesses. BUT, if we have tons of vaccinations when YOUNG, to ward off relatively minor diseases like measles, and mumps, etc.; we are setting ourselves up, since by compromising out immune systems and gut microbes to gain a perceived immunity to minor illnesses, we set ourselves up later for autoimmune diseases, cancer, and a host of really devastating diseases in our 50's and 60's, when we can't really fight them off.

And the modern vaccine? They are loaded with thimerosal, a mercury based preservative. And just the sheer AMOUNT of the stuff: twenty years ago children received 18 vaccines between 2 months and 5 years .

Now they receive 49 total vaccine doses between 2 months and 5 years and during this same twenty-year time frame (as we have increased the number of vaccines) we have seen a huge increase in autism, ADD/ADHD, allergies, asthma, and chronic illness that cannot be explained on environmental factors alone. Many call it coincidence. It is not.

Russia banned thimerosal from children's vaccines 20 years

195

ago, and Denmark, Austria, Japan, Great Britain and all the Scandinavian countries have since followed suit.

"You couldn't even construct a study that shows thimerosal is safe," says a Dr.Haley, who heads the chemistry department at the University of Kentucky. "It's just too darn toxic. If you inject thimerosal into an animal, its brain will sicken. If you apply it to living tissue, the cells die. If you put it in a petri dish, the culture dies. Knowing these things, it would be shocking if one could inject it into an infant without causing damage."

As Kelly Brogan, MD puts it: Ancestral health enthusiasts know that immunity cannot be manufactured, that buoying us with synthesized antibiotics and steroids — best left to emergency medicine — is a practice that is only necessitated by neglect of nutrition-based immune support.

When agencies point out that vaccines have greatly lowered death rates due to common diseases, you should know that the death rate by these diseases fell by over 90% before mass vaccinations began. Sanitation practices implemented at this time are the true cause of falling rates of disease. We should be thankful more to plumbers than to modern medicine!

Given all of the above, you probably think that I am totally anti-vaccine. No, but like most of modern medicine I think we have gotten carried away by progress and modernity, and abdicated responsibility for our own health and wellness to hospitals and clinics and doctors. The only one who can ensure your own health is YOU!

When human beings live according to their actual evolutionary biology, that is with God made foods of naturally raised animals and wild caught seafood, nuts, grass fed dairy, and organic vegetables and fruits, exercising and sleeping appropriately they tend to get really healthy. Humans that live in this natural, ancestral type of condition are very, very resistant to disease, because they are not chronically inflamed from huge amounts of man-made modern super gluten wheats and grains, rancid industrial seed oils like margarine and soy, and they have also preserved and help keep intact a thriving microbial population inside their guts! This last is incredibly important, as it is these gut microbes that keep us healthy and protect us from the many BAD microbes that are constantly working on infecting us.

But, since we do live in an age when disease is rampant- in addition, although this is hugely controversial just because it is politically incorrect, a time and place when mass illegal immigration from backwards countries is occurring, and exposing us to people who are carrying numerous diseases that heretofore were just about extinct in the developed world, I think a judicious, limited, and well spaced out choice of vaccines is ideal.

Get yourself a vaccine friendly pediatrician, one that really knows the pitfalls of the modern vaccine. Consider each vaccine carefully, and so SLOWLY as you give them, with plenty of recovery time between each one.

Here is one such plan, as laid out by the Wellness Mamma: Alternative Vaccination Schedule: Is There a Safe Way?

by The Paleo Mama
(This is the alternative vaccination schedule that is recommended by our vaccine-friendly Pediatrician.)

Alternative Vaccination Schedule (Select/Delay)
6 months DTaP (Diphtheria, Tetanus, and Pertussis)
9 months DTaP

12 months DtaP
15 months HIB (Haemophilus influenzae b)
18 months IPV (inactivated polio vaccine)
24 months IPV or Prevnar
27 months IPV or Prevnar
36 months MMR (measles, mumps, rubella)
48 months DTaP booster and IPV booster
5 years Whatever was not done at age 4.
Do not get the chicken pox vaccine, or the worse than
worthless Flu vaccine! And steer FAR clear of Gardasil!!
Unnecessary, and very dangerous!

Don't be one of those parents that feeds their kids cheeto's
and ding dongs, and buys them happy meals, and clears their
own conscience by "ensuring" their health with plenty of
vaccinations, medical visits, and medications!

 Give your kids a daily Paleo green smoothie made in your
Vitamix, go on family hikes, feed them bone broth,
homemade stews, and real, God made foods. These are the
greatest gifts you can give to your most precious possessions,
your children... and to yourself!

#

How to STAY Paleo

How to stay Paleo- eat a ton of veggies- All the rest is window
dressing!

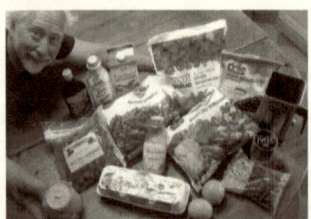

I know, this sounds like a vegan post, which I most definitely
am not. But, I stand by it.

198

PaleoJay's Smoothie Cafe!
* * *

If you start your day with a Paleo Green smoothie, loaded
with veggies and fruits, pre and probiotics, lots of good fat
and God made protein like free range eggs, your battle is
more than half won- drink a couple of good sized glasses
over the day, and you are already on track.

For one thing, you are quite full, and not vulnerable to be
tempted by bad fake food. For another "once begun- half
done" - the old truism is very true. Once you have started off
on the right foot, it is much, much easier to continue- have a
salad with some olive oil and vinegar, topped with meat and
hard boiled eggs for lunch, some nuts mid-afternoon, and
then (this is my ultimate deal sealer) grill a big juicy steak! (I
always try to grill bacon as well, which I can heat in the
morning with a few eggs- yum!)

The point is to always have lots of really good foods on hand-
ready to heat and eat, or just eat- then, temptation is easy to
resist.

Another thing- even though I live in a pretty rural area
(which I love!), even here we now have several places where
we can get things like sushi, and Vietnamese spring rolls.
 You can just pick them up, and you are set for a nutritious,
paleolithic meal instantly!

A good outdoor grill is a wonderful Paleo tool! I just got a
new, Weber charcoal grill (charcoal is vastly superior to gas-
use hardwood charcoal and you are in for wonderful foods).

My old grill is still functional; I set it back by our "tiny pub"
in the woods out back for parties and gatherings... it was
from the 1970's, so your investment lasts a long, long time!

Anyway, once or twice a week I shop for meats and veggies,

and load up that grill! Then, after an hour or so enjoying myself out by the grill, I have good, God made Paleo food for days, just heat and eat. Microwavable veggies are a perfect companion- I like to heat up butter at the same time as I do the veggies to top them off! Sometimes I am happy to just heat up two boxes of veggies, with butter, and that is my meal!

I think a real problem that folks have with staying Paleo is when they try to go too low carb. There definitely are advantages to going low carb, but low carb is not the same as no carb. Especially if you have a spouse that isn't really on board with the paleo diet, win them over by loading them up with LOTS of veggies (with butter and sea salt!), and also by having occasional sweet potato fries and loaded baked potatoes with sour cream, and even more butter! These "safe starches" will not hurt your health, especially if you work out they can even help you get healthier!

There is a place for really low carb; mostly for therapeutic uses as in the ketogenic diet- if you have an autoimmune disease, obesity, or conditions such as epilepsy, autism, alzheimer's, chron's disease, or diabetes- then a very, very low carb diet may be perfectly appropriate, even medicinal!

But for basically healthy, well folks: some safe starches will not impede your health, and may even enhance it! Have some fried rice with that beef and broccoli- just keep it in moderation!

The last thing I'd do to keep on keepin' paleo?

Listen to paleo podcasts. PaleoJay's Smoothie Cafe is one, and my other is Paleo Quick tip of the Day, both on iTunes and Stitcher. But Robb Wolf's the Paleo Solution is invaluable, as is Chris Kresser's Revolution Health Radio.

Latest in Paleo is another, as is Superhuman Radio with Carl Lenore... the advantage of listening to podcasts is that they reinforce, in a very personal, just me-to-you kind of informality, just what you are trying to do, why you are trying to do it, and just how really important it is to you in your life.

Oh- wait- one more thing!
STAY AWAY FROM MEDICAL DOCTORS, AND THEIR RECOMMENDATIONS!

This last is super important- medical clinics, hospitals, and the American Medical Association (along with their "trainers"- the pharmaceutical drug manufacturers, the FDA, and Monsanto itself) are totally invested in selling you as much bad, man engineered fake foods that destroy your health, and then selling you as many drugs as they can that mask the symptoms of your ruined health.

This is no illusion- follow the dollars!   There is so much money to be made if people are lured into eating processed foods in the selling of the foods that cause disease....

But there is even MORE money in selling the drugs to treat the diseases they cause!

Medical Doctors have pretty much been turned into drug pushers. And most commercials on TV are also drug pusher commercials!!
So- one more thing- avoid commercial TV!!
And it goes without saying: avoid drugs! Legal, illegal, it doesn't matter- and you know what? Illegal drugs are probably less harmful!!

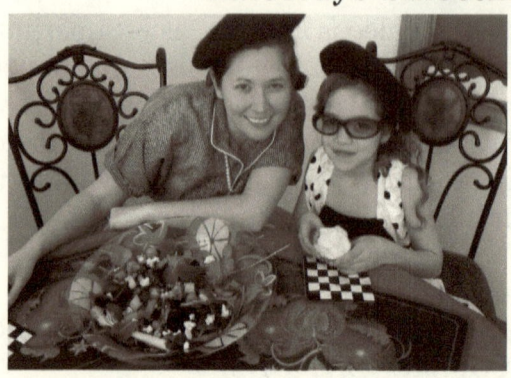

#

YOUR POLITICS DETERMINE YOUR NUTRITION

I have been thinking about this for quite some time, and think it's time to share. If you are a conservative or libertarian, I can probably tell just from that how you feed yourself and your family. Also, if you are a liberal, socialist or communist, that determines your views on nutrition and lifestyle as well.

Let's examine it, shall we? If you are on the left side of politics, there are certain near universal givens:

You believe that Big Government has most of the answers! You believe the top mainstream scientists, the big medical clinics, and the government agencies like the FDA, ADA, and all the rest have the peoples best interest well in hand, and are the "experts" that the American people should listen to, about everything- they are the smartest of the smart, and anyone who does not listen to them, and the AMA, and our industrial food supply experts is either stupid, selfish, or just

PaleoJay's Smoothie Cafe!

a "bitter clinger" that believes things were better in the past, when it is obvious to you that we are living in the best of times!

And so, given these viewpoints, you would tend to follow the USDA "My Plate" guidelines, which recommends multiple servings of grains per day, cutting fat out of the diet, reducing calories overall, and taking all sorts of drugs if your health markers are higher than your MD says is ideal as you go to your frequent medical appointments. You probably, if you exercise, go for long distances on treadmills at low intensity, perhaps for hours per day to "burn calories". And if you "jog" outdoors, you make sure to cover every inch of your body with sunscreen, as recommended by the Dermatologists! And you make sure to wear heavily padded shoes, to protect your feet from pounding.

You are happy to buy fat- free, highly processed foods like fruity yogurts at the grocery store, and enjoy lots of "healthy whole grains" in the form of breakfast cereals, granola bars, and whole grain bread (which of course you NEVER top with butter!) but instead with highly recommended vegetable oil margarine!

You cook with good fats like Crisco, and you stock up on plenty of good national brand orange juice and skimmed milk, since both are so healthy for you, as you've been told for your entire life by the government and the national media.

You are so glad that our water is kept fortified with fluoride, to strengthen our teeth, and are happy for all the chlorine and other chemicals which keeps it free of disease!

You probably also believe that putting statin drugs in the water as well would be a great preventive health measure,

203

and you support national control of school lunch programs.

And you LOVE it when your medical doctor (during one of your frequent "pr
eventive" appointments) recommends yet another drug for you to take- because, if he says you need it, well then you do! Now you will be healthy at last!

Now, let's say you are on the right- a libertarian or a true conservative...Pretty much everything is the opposite!

You believe in small, local government, and small local farms and ranches. You are very suspicious of the motives of large organizations, since as a rule they are all about making the maximum amount of money for themselves is a corporation, or gaining the maximum amount of power if they are a government agency.

You shop from locally owned stores, and prefer buying right from the farmer himself. The less processed the food is, the better it is! You completely reject the Governmental "My Plate", and have eliminated grains altogether from your diet.

You have added in real fats like pastured butter, eggs, and real cream and gotten rid of ALL fake vegetable oils. You drink real water, either filtered or good well water in preference to city treated stuff, and never drink bottled orange juice or skimmed milk, both of which are just basically sugar water which will spike your blood sugar, which then needs an emergency correction via insulin! You know better than to go down that road...

If you exercise, you work out short and intense, sprinting or working out with strength training at a very high level of exertion for short periods of time. If you sprint or run, you prefer doing it barefoot, and out in God's sunshine. You tan, but don't burn!

And there you have it! If you are paleo, you tend to be from on the right of things, a libertarian or conservative! Am I right? Leave me a message or comment- I am very interested in this take on the Paleo Lifestyle! Go to www.paleojay.com and leave a voice message on speakpipe there, or else just leave a written comment. I'll let you know the consensus!

The End of Strict Paleo!

ALCOHOL IS PALEO?

Did you know that alcohol was first probably found by our early ancestors in the form of fermented fruit hanging on or under trees or bushes, and was part of our diet at least 10 MILLION years ago! The common thought has been that alcohol was developed along with civilization roughly 10,000 years ago- not 10,000,000... but a scientist named Carrigan decided to settle the question by examining genetic evolution of the enzyme alcohol-ADH4 it's called. He then implanted this alcohol degrader into E.coli, and tested changes in the gene's sequence going back 70 million years.

The enzyme mimicking the enzyme as it was more long ago failed to metabolize alcohol- but at the 10 million year mark it worked fine! It worked just like the RDH4 lining our own guts- it's there to metabolize alcohol- just as it has been for 10 million years!

Now I'm not saying drinking alcohol is great- but I AM saying that it is a long standing real food choice of humans, and to eliminate it entirely is like eliminating something that is essentially part of the human condition. Always has been, always will be- one of the joys of being a man or woman, and a food source to boot...

Alcohol does NOT raise your insulin levels, although almost no governmental agency will admit it- just as they won't admit that eating 8-10 servings of grains per day WILL DRAMATICALLY raise your blood sugar, and hence insulin levels! In fact, alcohol can actually increase your insulin

206

sensitivity.

 Moderate alcohol consumption improves insulin sensitivity, lowers triglyceride concentrations and improves glycemic control. Not only in healthy folks, but also in type 2 diabetes. There is no clear consensus on the insulin sensitizing mechanism of alcohol, but one viable explanation may be that alcohol promotes leanness by stimulating AMPK in skeletal muscle. It's not a stretch to assume that this might have favorable effects on nutrient partitioning in the longer term.

If the effect of alcohol consumption on insulin sensitivity doesn't impress you, then consider the fact that studies have consistently shown that moderate drinkers live longer than non-drinkers. This can be mainly attributed to a lowered risk of cardiovascular disease. However, alcohol also contributes to a healthier and disease-free life by protecting against Alzheimer's disease, metabolic syndrome, rheumatoid arthritis, the common cold, different types of cancers, depression and many other Western diseases. The list goes on and on.

It can almost be said beyond doubt that moderate alcohol consumption is healthier than complete abstinence. With this in mind, it's strange that the fitness and health community shun alcohol. This irrational attitude seems to be grounded in the beliefs that alcohol is fattening and will hamper muscle gains.

And to really muddy the waters: even beer seems to be OK for non-celiacs! At least in my case, (I am not celiac), although I avoid gluten at every juncture in the eating of food, in beer it really does not seem to matter- especially if you confine yourself to blonde, Pilsner types of beers- and especially if you drink the low end, cheap commercial beers made of corn and rice!!

And not just Budweiser, but all of those really low end, American beers, like Hamm's, and Blatz, and Coors and Corona (not really low end there, but you get the idea!).

And here is a quote from the Heinekin's website:

"Beer contains gluten, which comes from the grain from which it is brewed. Only a fraction of the gluten that the grain contains gets into the beer. The proportion depends on the kind of grain that is used. The use of barley results only in traces of gluten in the beer whilst wheat contributes considerably more. It also depends on the brewing process. Generally speaking: the clearer and blonder the beer is, the less gluten it may contain. Some people are allergic to gluten and have to follow a diet that minimises or excludes their gluten intake. Whether beer can be part of such a diet or not, is dependent on the extent of the allergy and the beer type consumed. In many cases lager beers pose no problem for people who have a gluten allergy. However, it is up to the individual to assess his or her sensitivity."

Bottom line?

If you want to be really healthy, a Paleo superhuman for a long and healthy life, I would eliminate gluten as early as possible from my diet. The less gluten the better, and this increases the older you get- the insult to the gut lining just multiplies, and you set yourself up for autoimmunity, obesity, and diabesity more and more and more- so just stop! PLEASE!!

And so far as the indulgence of alcoholic libations, they are OK within reason, and nothing when compared to the unfiltered, huge amounts of horrid gluten held in the many fast and processed foods most folks deem to hold so harmless. They are in actuality far worse than cigarette smoking, and will give you a slow, lingering death worse than lung cancer or heart disease in all likelihood...

So drink up instead! If you eliminate food sources of gluten, and severely limit carbs as well- you will get slim and healthy, and feel great! AND, you will most likely NOT become celiac, and so can continue to feel great, stay slim and healthy, and not have to worry about having to eliminate the "small" sources of gluten, like beer, that contains about 20 parts per million in light, or blonde lager beers.

There is something about the fermentation process itself that is self protective to us, since the yeast consumes all the sugars, whatever the source, and alters the grain sources so much that they become much less harmful.

This is one of those facts that seem to be hard to find, since they are so politically incorrect.

PROSIT!

www.ingramcontent.com/pod-product-compliance
Lightning Source LLC
Chambersburg PA
CBHW050442290526
45786CB00006B/2130